1995

The

ROLE

of the

PHYSICIAN

EXECUTIVE

The
ROLE
of the
PHYSICIAN
EXECUTIVE
Cases and
Commentary

Edited by
DAVID A. KINDIG
ANTHONY R. KOVNER

with the editorial assistance of
Beverly Hills and Mary Schuster

Health Administration Press
Ann Arbor, Michigan   1992

The cases in this book are based on actual situations, but they have been fictionalized in the interests of the participants. The editors gratefully acknowledge the help and support of the hospitals and health facilities involved.

96 95 94 93 92   5 4 3 2 1

Library of Congress Cataloging-in-Publication Data

The Role of the physician executive : cases and commentary / edited by
David A. Kindig and Anthony R. Kovner with the editorial assistance of Beverly
Hills and Mary Schuster.
    p.   cm.
    Includes bibliographical references.
    ISBN 0-910701-88-2 (softbound : alk. paper)
    1. Health services administration—Case studies.   2. Physician executives—
Case studies.   I. Kindig, David A.   II. Kovner, Anthony.
    [DNLM: 1. Health Facilities—organization & administration.   2. Health
Facility Administrators.   3. Physician's Role.   WX 155 R745]
RA971.R563   1992   362.a'1'068—dc20
DNLM/DLC for Library of Congress   92-49823 CIP

The paper used in this publication meets the minimum requirements of American National Standard for Information Sciences—Permanence of Paper for Printed Library Materials, ANSI Z39.48-1984. ⊚ ™

Health Administration Press
A division of the Foundation of the
   American College of Healthcare Executives
1021 East Huron Street
Ann Arbor, Michigan 48104-9990
(313) 764-1380

Contents

Foreword

This exceptional work is a welcome and exciting contribution to the emerging specialty of medical management and, indeed, to all of health care administration.

In the past, there has been much speculation—albeit somewhat intuitive and anecdotal—about the contribution that physicians trained in management could make to the leadership and administration of health care organizations. It has been said that physicians who could span the boundaries—in language, skill, ethics, and values—between medicine and management could play a critical role in more effectively integrating the clinical and administrative systems in an organization. Thus far, however, this boundary-spanning role has been discussed only in the abstract. There has been little documentation of real-life examples in which firsthand knowledge of both the clinical process and the managerial process has made a difference. The superbly written cases presented in this book begin to show concretely how the ability to span system boundaries might lead to more effective management in health care organizations.

This book also makes an important contribution to the effort to bridge the gap between clinical and managerial training. For 15 years, I have watched physicians struggle with the lack of "how to's" in their managerial education. This book uses a case method that is familiar to physicians and that closely represents the managerial job that the physician executive is being asked to do. The cases require the integration of data and disciplines, they contain uncertainties, and they allow for the consideration of personalities and policies.

Finally, the editors and authors of this book have made another contribution to health services administration, which may be less apparent, but is no less significant. Many physicians have been turning from clinical practice to management. Fortunately, most do so to make positive changes in the evolution of their organizations or to have a greater influence on health care systems. Unfortunately, however, many physicians are running from clinical practice without a true picture of the nature of managerial work—its demands, anxieties, and challenges, and the training required to do an effective job. If this book does nothing other than to give lay physicians some insight into the actual demands and skills required of physician executives, it will still have done a great service to the profession.

Roger Schenke
American College of Physician Executives

Preface

This book of cases and commentary is written for physician executives, for those who wish to be physician executives, and for those who wish to teach physician executives. The book is a compilation of 19 recent managerial case studies involving physician executives. The cases examine the following issues that confront physician executives:

- Unnecessary surgery and overutilization of hospital services by physicians
- Physician/hospital ownership of services and pursuit of joint programs
- Paying physicians
- Setting management priorities
- Merging and governing combined clinical departments and HMOs
- Emergency department overcrowding
- State government judicial rulings affecting medical practice
- Social and quality-of-care issues for low-income populations

Physician executives can use this book to gain an understanding of how other physician executives address similar problems and to learn about the ways in which a physician executive's job is and is not unique. Local circumstances vary, but strategies for effectively managing physician behavior may be similar.

Physicians who are considering becoming executives will find that this book will help them determine whether or not they indeed wish to take on the challenges and constraints facing physician executives. Several different work settings and contexts—including hospitals, nursing homes, HMOs, government, and group practices—are described in the book. Finally, those wishing to teach physician executives can use this book as a textbook in their health administration courses. The two appendixes to the book explore the case method approach to teaching and its relevance to the study of health services administration. Most of the cases have been tested in the classroom, and the teaching notes give suggestions for classroom use. We urge you and others to write your own management cases for teaching physician executives. David Kindig and I are available to help you in this effort.

Anthony R. Kovner, Ph.D.
New York University
Robert F. Wagner Graduate School of Public Service

Part I

Introduction: Two Views of the New Physician Executive

Physician Executives: A Dual Role Emerges

David A. Kindig, M.D.

The past five years have seen a marked increase in the amount of attention paid to the part physicians play in the management of health care organizations. Journals regularly feature this topic. The American College of Physician Executives (ACPE) is growing rapidly, sponsoring a certification examination, and seeking recognition as the representative of a legitimate medical specialty. The Association of University Programs in Health Administration devoted its 1988 plenary session to "Management Education for the Physician Executive." And executive search firms report increased requests for physician executives. There is even some concern that physicians trained primarily in administration may replace their clinically trained counterparts in many senior positions in health care organizations.

What is a physician executive? The terms "physician administrator," "clinician administrator," "physician executive," and "physician manager" are often used interchangeably. Detmer[1] distinguishes between the "physician manager," a full-time executive without clinical responsibilities, and the "clinician executive," who acts as both administrator and clinician. "Physician executive" is used here because the "clinician executive" category includes nurses, dentists, and other non-physicians. Individuals who no longer engage in clinical practice

Reprinted from *Decisions in Imaging Economics* 3, no. 4 (1990): 30–34, with permission, *Decisions in Imaging Economics*.

are included as physician executives, since many still make active use of their clinical knowledge. Excluded from the category are MDs whose administrative responsibilities involve no clinical expertise and practicing physicians whose administrative functions require only minor amounts of time. American College of Physician Executives fellowship requirements (board certification in a clinical specialty, substantial clinical practice experience, expanding managerial responsibility, and demonstrated managerial knowledge) best define the term "physician executive."

Over the past several years, we have performed many studies on physicians regarding executive roles. For research purposes, we defined "physician executives" as those MDs listed in the American Medical Association's Physician Masterfile whose primary professional activity, as measured by self-reported hours worked per week, is administration. In 1985, this group consisted of 13,500 individuals, or 3 percent of physicians listed in the Masterfile as active in patient care. Some of their basic characteristics, compiled from information collected during telephone interviews conducted by the Wisconsin Survey Research Laboratory on a sample of 878 of these physicians,[2] are shown in Table 1.

Additional findings indicate that their reasons for choosing management work were largely activist, such as "desire to impact health care delivery and quality of care" and preference for "new opportunities and challenges." Traditional views of administration as a preretirement activity or as an act of personal sacrifice—"someone needs to do it"—were rarely cited. Seventy-five percent of the respondents predicted that the need for physician executives will grow because the more complex business orientation of the health care system, as well as mounting political pressures and governmental control efforts, mandates greater physician involvement in administrative decisions.

While only 3 percent of the 878 physicians held graduate management degrees other than the MPH (master of public health) degree held by 9.8 percent, 84 percent felt that management degrees are advisable. Of the physician executives who participated in the study, 517 also completed a managerial task inventory[3] consisting of 33 tasks in five categories (see Table 2). Other studies have indicated that physician executives' responsibilities usually concern the management of other physicians and emphasize staff supervision, medical education, and quality assurance duties. In our findings, however, governance and internal management tasks were nearly as important and time-consuming as clinical internal management and were ranked as much more important than the supervision of physicians.

This confirms that the physician executive's managerial duties encompass general administration as well as clinical/physician manage-

Table 1 Characteristics of Physician Executives—1986

Characteristic	Response
Average age	54.2 years
Average years in administration	18.6 years
Average number of previous administrative positions	2.3 positions
Average years in current administrative position	7.2 years
Average number of hours worked	54.2 hours per week
Percentage of time in administration	64.9%
Percentage of time in patient care	20.5%
Mean total annual income	$110,300
Type of organization	
Hospital	30%
Educational institute	24%
Government agency	23%
Group practice/HMO	5%
Health care corporation	5%
Industry	4%
Other	8%

Source: Responses to a telephone survey from 878 physicians whose self-reported primary professional activity was administration in the 1985 American Medical Association Physician Masterfile.

Table 2 Physician Executive Role—Mean Rank of 33 Tasks by Category: Importance and Time Spent per Week

Clinical internal management	10.4
Governance	12.5
General internal management	13.4
External activities	20.3
Management of physicians	23.0

Source: Response to a task survey by 519 physician executives drawn from the telephone survey sample presented in Table 1.

ment activities and constitute a boundary-spanning role. Many tasks in the external activity category were ranked as "not done but should be," including "working to change regulations and legislation" and "generating philanthropic support." Internal tasks in the same group of necessary but neglected items included "evaluating physician performance regarding costs" and "dealing with physician burnout/impairment."

Examination of the career development of physicians in management revealed that career moves, whether between institutions or between different types of health care organizations, were made less frequently by physician executives than by other health care executives. Physician executives, however, change their affiliations much more frequently than practicing clinicians do. Sixty percent of respondents had worked in only one type of health care organization; of these, 57 percent had spent their entire managerial careers employed by one institution.[4] Sixteen percent of the 878 respondents held senior titles such as CEO/ president, dean, or surgeon general. The highest seniority percentage, 23 percent, was found among those who had worked in two different types of health care organizations, perhaps indicating recognition for the value of experience gained in varying settings.

Another of our objectives was analysis of the total time spent in managerial pursuits (other than practice management) and how this amount had changed over the previous decade. The AMA Masterfile's hours per week data were used to compare activity in the primary and secondary/tertiary categories.[5] As shown in Table 3, the largest time increases have occurred in secondary/tertiary management, with 30 percent growth in the number of physicians involved and a 14 percent increase in hours required. Overall, the number of full-time equivalents (FTEs) devoted to management has grown 38 percent in ten years. The largest increases in time expenditure are seen among physicians under the age of 45.

Management education for physician executives is often incomplete. Of physicians whose principal activity was management, 12.7 percent reported holding a management master's degree; 9.8 percent of these degrees, however, were MPH degrees awarded an average of 17 years before the survey was conducted. Such degree programs probably did not provide management education as it is currently understood. The remaining 2.9 percent of the management degrees reported were master of business administration (MBA) and master of science (MS) degrees awarded within eight and 11 years, respectively, which would probably have more in common with current management training. The educational attainments of physicians who had only secondary/ tertiary management duties were not investigated.

In 1989, Grebenschikoff and Kirschman[6] reported on a salary survey involving 1,200 ACPE members. Of the hospital-based physician executives in this sample, 15.7 percent held advanced degrees, of which 3 percent were MBAs, 3 percent were MPHs, 1.2 percent were MHAs (master of health administration), and 5.2 percent were MSs. An additional 10.4 percent reported working toward a degree. Health maintenance organization (HMO) executives held the highest percentage of MBA and MS degrees. In a larger sample from the AMA Masterfile, 22 percent of respondents felt that formal graduate course work or an

Table 3 Number of Physicians, Average Number of Hours Worked
per Week in Administration, and Number of FTEs as a
Primary or Secondary/Tertiary Activity, 1977 and 1986

	Number of Physicians		
	1977	1986	% Change
Primary Activity	11,800	14,075	19.2
Secondary/Tertiary Activity	129,083	168,387	30.4
	Average Hours Worked per Week		
	1977	1986	% Change
Primary Activity	34.3	33.7	−1.2
Secondary/Tertiary Activity	5.7	6.5	14.0
	Number of FTEs		
	1977	1986	% Change
Primary Activity	7,092	8,345	17.7
Secondary/Tertiary Activity	13,002	19,290	48.4

Source: Kindig D, Dunham N: How much administration is today's physician doing?
Physician Executive, 1990; 17(1): 3–7.

advanced degree would be required of future physician executives, and
62 percent indicated that such training would be advisable.

Given these findings, how should medical managers decide on the
type and amount of advanced management education to obtain? Degree
considerations should not always take priority, as the pursuit of a formal graduate degree is an expensive and time-consuming process. For
those who have little or no management experience, part-time administrative activity is a simpler way to gain preliminary exposure to management. The ACPE's "Physician in Management" seminars also are an
excellent introduction and should be attended preceding serious consideration of a graduate degree. Similarly, workshops or individual courses
covering accounting, health law, or quality assurance may satisfy immediate knowledge requirements.

After completing these initial steps, many individuals commit
themselves to a career in medical management and plan to obtain a
management master's degree. Their reasons usually combine two factors: either the course work required for immediate needs is nearly as
substantial as that required to obtain a degree or gaining a degree is
expected to enhance career advancement and recognition. Greben-

schikoff and Kirschman conclude that an advanced degree is not critical in the selection of physician executives; experience, for example, may carry greater importance. Other factors being equal, however, an advanced degree may provide a candidate with an advantage in obtaining a particular position. Within five to eight years, some sort of formal management degree will probably be expected by most health care organizations.

Any predictions that can be made for the future of medical management include more questions than answers. Will demand for physician executives increase? Will this demand eradicate the physician surplus predicted for the coming century, as one investigator claims? How will the physician executive's role change, and how will it relate to the roles of other health care executives? How will other clinician executives, such as nurses, interact with physician executives? Will physician executives use their increasing knowledge of management methods to seek professional dominance, or will they adopt a team management approach? Will health care organizations employing physician executives demonstrate gains in the quality, appropriateness, efficiency, or empathy of the care they provide? Will a credentialing mechanism be developed for physician executives? If so, will it give employers a reliable measure of the individual's physician executive potential?

Questions concerning the education of physician executives are nearly as numerous. Is a graduate degree required, or can sufficient knowledge be gained through individual courses and seminars? Is management education best conducted during medical school and residency, or is it more effective after a period of clinical practice? Are existing MHA or MBA degree programs appropriate, or will physician executives need a modified curriculum? What academic content should such curricula provide? Is graduate education for physician executives more effectively presented in classes reserved for MDs, or should other students be included? What educational format or technology is appropriate for adult learners near the peak of their careers?

Though questions will continue to abound, some answers can be proposed with relative certainty. The physician executive's role will grow in importance as the crisis of cost continues to dominate health care. Physicians will not replace nonclinicians as CEOs in large numbers, but physicians and nurses who have administrative experience will compete more vigorously for such positions. Most importantly, these executives will bring important skills and knowledge to the leadership team, enabling their employers to perform more efficiently.

There are three reasons that these predictions can be made confidently. First, excellence in organizational leadership requires solid grounding in substance. Though many senior health care executives who are not physicians have gained considerable familiarity with clinical issues, competitive business pressures will not allow their younger colleagues sufficient time to develop such skills. Even if their duties required less time, new administrators would be unable to obtain the experience physician executives acquire through years of direct patient care. For "knowledge of the business," health care organizations will need clinicians who can integrate practice and management.

Second, as Ellwood[7] states, "medical management is a clinical science." He delineates five areas in which health care organizations must possess expertise if they are to reduce costs and improve care: health management, medical management information systems, medical decision theory, sociology/psychology of organized medical care, and health promotion/disease prevention. The physician or nurse executive is in an excellent position to bring this necessary expertise to the executive suite.

Third, executives who have clinical experience transport their professional values and ethics into health care management. Biomedical ethics issues will continue to be important, and clinicians can bring greater understanding of these problems to the corporate level. Their concerns will naturally be incorporated in their general managerial ethics. Responsibility for the individual patient's welfare, a guiding ethic for most clinicians, will allow physician executives to apply an augmented "conscience" at the organizational level.

In summary, the importance of the physician executive will continue to grow. Many future physician executives will hold modern master's degrees in health management; most will fill boundary-spanning roles emphasizing clinical management science. Some will compete successfully for CEO positions. The emergence of a stronger role for physician executives will require changes in the structure of the management team, but health care organizations that are able to make the necessary adjustments will be rewarded with better performance in both cost control and quality improvement.

Notes

1. Detmer DE: The physician as corporate practitioner and corporate leader. Presented July 31, 1984. *Duke University National Forum on Hospital and Health Affairs,* 56–64.
2. Kindig DA, Lastiri-Quiros S: Administrative medicine: A new specialty? *Health Affairs,* Winter 1986; 146–156.
3. Kindig DA, Lastiri-Quiros S: The changing managerial role of physician executives. *The Journal of Health Administration Education,* 1989; 7(1): 33–46.

4. Kindig D, Dunham N, Man-Chun L: Career paths of physician executives. *Health Care Management Review*, 1991; 16(4): 11–20.
5. Kindig D, Dunham N: How much administration is today's physician doing? *Physician Executive*, 1990; 17(1): 3–7.
6. Grebenschikoff J, Kirschman D: Getting the third degree. *Physician Executive*, 1989; 15(2): 27–28.
7. In conversation with Paul Ellwood, 1989.

The Dual Role Dilemma

Michael E. Kurtz

While physicians bring unique characteristics to the managerial role, they are also unique products of the culture of the medical profession. They have made major personal commitments to a profession and a career very early in life, and the professional culture they enter definitely shapes their values, beliefs, ideas, internal and external perceptions, behaviors, and personalities.

Physicians spend the most formative years of their professional lives almost exclusively in the company of other physicians (teachers, mentors, preceptors, etc.) and the professional values and norms of the world of medicine are strongly inculcated and reinforced on a daily basis. Also, for a physician to be successful in the clinical role and to achieve acceptance and recognition from the medical community, he or she must be willing to accept and demonstrate these values and norms; otherwise the physician will find him- or herself treated as an unacceptable member of the community and severely criticized. To be able to pass through the ranks, rites of passage, and hierarchy of the medical community, one must be willing to comply and behave in accordance with these norms and expectations.

This socialization process of the "becoming-physician" probably has more direct influence on behaviors exhibited later in practice than

Reprinted from *The Physician Executive*, edited by W. Curry (Tampa, FL: American College of Physician Executives, 1988), with permission, American College of Physician Executives.

anything else. Upon examination, I have found that although most physicians share similar values, have experienced similar initial training, and identify as a distinct professional group, the individual specialties of medicine provide further socialization, demand specialty identification, and develop unique behavioral characteristics within their subgroups.

When analyzed through a series of behavior-oriented assessments, each specialty is found to use behaviors that are unique and specific to it; i.e., most surgeons act and behave as other surgeons, most pediatricians act and behave as other pediatricians, etc. These behaviors (whether successful or unsuccessful in achieving the individual's goals) are reinforced by other members of the physician's primary identification group and are constantly rewarded and reinforced in the clinical setting.

In general, most physicians (i.e., all specialists) are oriented to certain behaviors and values in their clinical practices, and these behaviors are successful for them and most likely are needed if they are to achieve the desired outcomes and acceptance of colleagues and peers.

When the physician moves away from the clinical role and into the world of management, administration, and leadership, we find that he/she most often will continue to use these learned clinical behaviors, professional norms, and values. A negative result is seen when this occurs. While clinical behaviors are critical for success in the practitioner role, they tend to create conflict, resistance, and tension in the managerial role.

Through an ongoing study, a long list of differences between effective clinicians and effective managers has been defined. When factored to determine those that are most critical, a list of nine major differences emerges (see below).

Major Differences between Clinicians and Managers

Clinicians	Managers
Doers	Planners, designers
1:1 interactions	1:N interactions
Reactive personalities	Proactive personalities
Require immediate gratification	Accept delayed gratification
Deciders	Delegators
Value autonomy	Value collaboration
Independent	Participative
Patient advocate	Organization advocate
Identify with profession	Identify with organization

Clinicians are action oriented. They are "doers" and hands-on oriented. They prefer to be directly involved in their work, and see themselves as the primary interacters in most situations (e.g., diagnostic workups, treatment, etc.). Managers, on the other hand, see their primary role as being in planning and designing. Managers work through a process that establishes goals and objectives, and then facilitate the planning and designing of activities that will accomplish these goals. They are not "doers"—that role is delegated to staff. Once you become a "doer," you are a worker, not a manager. When clinicians actively participate in the work itself, they are most often seen as interfering in organization operations.

Clinicians feel most effective, and report feeling most comfortable and most successful, in one-to-one encounters and interactions. They prefer to deal with others on an individual basis, whether this be doctor/patient, doctor/nurse, doctor/family, doctor/doctor, etc. In a study of 800 physician-managers, I found that they tended to be very selective in the groups they join. They preferred to be left alone and were somewhat detached, independent, and self-sufficient. They demonstrated low interest in being included by others (especially in social activities) and had little concern about prestige or what others thought. (This may be a result of the medical training process, which traditionally prepares physicians for solo practice and for orientation to the private doctor/patient relationship.)

This low inclusion behavior may prove to be successful for the medical practitioner, but it lowers effectiveness for the physician-manager. The managerial role demands a high degree of group interaction in the organizational setting in order to accomplish effective decision-making and problem-solving and, where appropriate, to establish participative and collaborative team management. Approximately 73 percent of a manager's time is spent in meetings and group settings. Physicians find these situations (i.e., meetings) intolerable and perceive them as a waste of time.

Clinicians are trained as reactive personalities. They are inclined to wait for their clinical services to be needed and/or requested. The physician waits for the patient to present himself, or to be referred; the physician most often responds to a need already defined and/or in progress. To be effective in management, the individual must work from a proactive stance, which means that the manager must anticipate future needs and requirements and initiate and/or invent processes to address them.

Obtaining short-term and/or immediate results/gratification is reported as being extremely important to the physician, who desires to quickly see a result from taking an action or initiating an intervention and experiences frustration when this is not realized. Managers very seldom experience immediate results from their work. Because they most often work in planning and designing processes, anticipating future events, etc., they are forced to accept delayed results/gratification for the investment of their energies. A manager may not see the result of his or her work for months or even years (anyone who has been involved in a building project can easily understand this dynamic).

Physicians are trained to be independent problem-solvers and perceive themselves to be the deciders in almost all medical/clinical decision situations. They see themselves as having the ultimate authority and responsibility, and they will almost always assume this role and display this behavior. While managers have the "right" of decision-making and reserve the "right to veto," they will most often delegate decision-making to their subordinates. As stated above, organization leaders *manage the process* of problem solving and decision-making. To always be the deciders would place them in a position of being perceived as autocratic, authoritarian, and mistrusting of their subordinates. Also, it is important to recognize that with the high degree of specialization and subspecialization that has evolved and developed in both the clinical and managerial fields, no one person can be expected to have all of the expertise and/or knowledge required for complex decision-making. Multiple resources will always be required.

The perception of being the "decider" held by the physician is further reinforced by the clinician's value of autonomy. Physicians tend to see themselves as autonomous professionals whose responsibility is to their patients and their profession. They are the ones to determine their level of involvement and interaction, and they don't perceive themselves to be subordinate or subservient to others. They prefer to perform their roles independently and autonomously, only involving others as they determine. While this value of autonomy protects the clinician from being politically influenced, it can significantly interfere with his or her effectiveness in a leadership/managerial role. Managers cannot function autonomously by the very nature of the definition of their role and function. Managers value collaboration and integration. They see their primary function as being one of facilitating and supporting the merging of ideas through the collaboration of organizational functions and related personnel. The actions of any one part of the organization affect every other part of the organization. Therefore, shared information, integration of ideas and resources, and collaboration of team members with other managers are absolutely requisite in maximizing the larger whole (i.e., reaching the goals and objectives of the organization). All decision-making and problem-solving must be entered into with the orientation of what will be best for the greater good (of the organization) rather than what will be best for the individual. The value of autonomy held by most physicians results in a fairly high degree of self-centeredness and is often perceived as selfishness by nonclinical members of the organization.

Concomitant with the value of autonomy is the value of independence held by the clinician. Physicians are trained to work independently, to make independent decisions, and to take independent responsibility for outcomes. They don't want to feel that they are dependent on others for the successes or the failures they experience. Research data demonstrate [that physicians have] a very low need for inclusion of and involvement by others, a low need to participate with others in situations that don't directly affect them, and a relatively high need to take charge. Physicians enjoy making decisions and influencing others and resist allowing others to influence them. They don't want others (especially nonphysicians) to tell them what to do, and they consume a great deal of physical and psychological energy protecting this autonomy and independence.

Concomitant with the value of collaboration, managers strongly value participation and avoid independent behaviors and actions. To ensure quality and commitment in decision-making and problem-solving, managers recognize the need to involve others in the process. They see their role as one of facilitating and supporting the involvement and participation of others in order to obtain maximum synergism. An effective manager is a person who designs and plans an organizational system that creates a culture and environment that encourages and supports participation by all members of the organization and one that discourages independence and ivory tower decision-making.

Another major difference between clinicians and managers is that the physician assumes the primary role of being an advocate for the patient. Physicians assume the responsibility of protecting the patients from undue outside influence and interference. In many cases, the outside influence is defined as the organization and the management and administrative system. Clinicians are oriented to the concept that, "if the patient needs something, one gets it for him." To be asked to do cost-benefit analysis, or to be told that certain interventions or services are inappropriate, is untenable to a clinician, and is seen as interfering with professional prerogatives and responsibilities.

While managers are not insensitive to patient needs and to an acceptable level of quality in patient care, they are required to primarily function as advocates of the organization. The manager's role, function, and responsibility require that he or she work to enhance and build the organization as a whole and to maximize its efficiency, productivity, and assets. When working with others, managers do not represent themselves; they function as representatives and advocates of the organization. The manager will constantly be striving to ensure viability of the organization, and, therefore, decisions will be made that will be in the best interest of the larger whole rather than in the interest of individuals. Clinicians will often make decisions based on isolated, unique, and specific facts of a certain case that may appear (or be) inconsistent with decisions made in related cases. Managers, on the other hand, are expected to make decisions that are consistent with organization policy, values, and norms. This concept of consistency and predictability carries extreme weight in evaluating effective managerial behavior, otherwise the manager would be managing by exception to the rule, which would result in organizational chaos.

This difference in advocacy orientation is further exaggerated by the individual's identification with a professional group or organizational entity. Physicians identify with their professional group and, more specifically, with their specialization within the larger professional designation. When asked "who are you," a clinician will first respond that he or she is a physician and then further define this identity with his or her specialization. The next level of identification is most often as a member of a certain medical community or communities (e.g., XYZ Hospital medical staff, ABC Physicians, or as a recognized member of several different hospital medical staffs within a community). The very last identification will be as a manager, administrator, or as a representative of a specific organization. The clinician identifies with the organization only insofar as it allows the practice of skill and demonstration of the clinician's expertise. Physicians do not relate to the concept of "employment" or "unemployment." They perceive themselves as being able to practice wherever and whenever they choose. Because of that orientation, the physician sees the organization as simply a place that provides the opportunity, facilities, and environment to "practice," and this place could actually be anywhere.

The manager is in quite a different situation; his or her identity is totally dependent on employment or unemployment by an organization. Therefore, the identification is with the organization and not the professional field. Without an organization to manage, the manager can no longer be identified as a manager. Managers derive satisfaction from the rewards given and by the value accorded by the organization, which, in turn, affords recognition and acceptance by the larger managerial community. When asked the same question, "Who are you?", the manager will respond that he or she is the chief executive officer or the manager/director of the computer sciences department of XYZ Health Center. The manager perceives him- or herself as "belonging" to the

XYZ Health Center, and the organization provides, promotes, and dictates this identification. The manager's role and responsibility is to develop the organization and to protect its viability in the marketplace, which creates competitive behavior and further fosters the identification with "us." This feeling of "my country, right or wrong" is totally foreign to the clinician when translated to the organization context.

These differences between clinicians and managers are but a few in a long list of practical and philosophical differences, but they are the major ones and they tend to create the greatest degree of role-conflict and dual role dilemma for the physician-manager. It is important to recognize that each set of behaviors, practices, and skills is necessary for satisfactory performance in the specific role demand (i.e., clinician or manager), but the physician who chooses to enter into management and administration will most often find him- or herself straddling the chasm between the two.

Most physician-managers feel that it is important to maintain a clinical involvement, and there is a strong argument for this. The clinician wishes to at least maintain, if not enhance, clinical skills and abilities, to learn and update knowledge and skills from participation and interaction with colleagues, and to continue identification with the medical community and specialty. The clinician has spent the major part of his or her adult life in this community and has developed almost an exclusive identity with it. To leave it and move into another "profession" and career path is a psychologically wrenching and threatening experience. It means turning one's back on the primary identification group, giving up membership in an exclusive and elite professional "club," and starting out on a new educational and professional road. This choice requires leaving an area of acquired personal and professional expertise and recognition that is very comfortable and highly rewarded and moving into a relatively uncomfortable area with little, if any, preparation. It demands leaving an area of recognized professional competence and moving into the role of neophyte, learner, and student. This shift, along with the basic negative attitudes and perceptions about managers held by most physicians, further feeds the role-conflict and dual role dilemma for the clinician.

There is another identity issue that emerges for the physician-manager. Along with the personal identity dilemma is the question of identification that is raised for the medical community and the organization membership. The physician can never rid him- or herself of the title of "Doctor" and will always be perceived as a physician by the organization's membership. The clinician will always be one of "them" in the eyes of nonphysician executives and staff, and, historically and through training and experience, "them" has always been an adversarial group. Therefore, the physician executive's allegiances, commitment, and dedication will always be questioned.

At the same time, the medical staff and/or community will now perceive its colleague as a member of the management and administrative staff, which has always been a "them" to that group. This is especially true if the physician-manager is employed and paid by the organization and may lead to questioning and mistrust of communication and intent.

Some physicians and management experts will argue that it is impossible to maintain this dual role—that one cannot adequately and competently perform in one while also practicing the other. The concern of becoming a "Jack of all trades, master of none" is a very real one and must be addressed by the professional community as well as the organization. With the strong movement to "professionalize" the role of physician-manager/physician-executive taking place in the United States, it can be assumed that this role will require certification of competence and capability in the very near future and that this "certification" will require demonstration of education, training, skill development, and experience in managerial roles and responsibilities. No longer can the physician simply assume an organizational leadership or management role because he or she is a good clinician; these successful clinician skills and behaviors are being recognized as creating problems in the practice of management and administration. A shift in thinking, philosophy, attitudes, and behavior must take place if the physician is to be seen as successful and as an asset to the organization.

I don't think that it must necessarily be an either/or question. Experience demonstrates that those physician-executives who are recognized as the most competent, capable, and successful have, through their own choices and the demands of their organizations, given up clinical involvement and have dedicated themselves to the professionalization of the physician-executive role. They have not lost credibility with their medical colleagues because they have developed competence and expertise as managers. They are perceived as being sensitive to the needs and values of the medical community while being accorded credibility through the quality and fairness of their decisions and human relations skills. Their organizations tend to be large and complex, which requires full-time commitment and dedication to the managerial role. They also tend to be organizations that are physician-owned and/or physician-run, so that the entire medical staff is in some way involved in the management of the organization.

It is probably not an either/or question; it is more a factor of the size and the complexity of the organization that will provide the answer.

A 15-person medical group can't afford to have one of its physicians excluded from a clinical role, but a 60+ person group can't afford not to force the choice if it desires adequate and successful management.

I don't think that this dual role dilemma can be easily resolved for the physician-manager. It will require some soul-searching, self-analysis, and the development of self-awareness for each individual. For the physician to be successful in the dual role requires that he or she thoroughly understand which hat is being worn at which time, be adequately prepared for each in order to obtain and maintain credibility, and make sure that those people working for and with the physician executive understand which hat is being worn at any specific time.

It's also important for the physician-manager to use this unique position to develop and enhance collaboration and integration of the medical and administrative staffs in the daily management and operations of the organization. Through this mechanism, the chasm of the dual roles and its concomitant frustration and conflict can be bridged.

Health care organizations are struggling with a rapidly changing economic, political, and social environment. Many are developing successful new businesses and service strategies, while others are suffering failure. It is predicted that 20–25 percent of currently operating hospitals will close within the next two to three years, and 30–40 percent of health care providers other than hospitals (e.g., clinics, group practices, HMOs, etc.) will initiate major organizational restructuring, redesign, and redefinition, or be the targets of takeovers and mergers.

Upon reviewing more than 60 such situations, I found that, although various strategies are being tested, there has been one underlying theme that emerges: the activities of the most responsive and strongest health care organizations all, in some way, support the integration of their medical staffs into the operational management and leadership of the organization.

The traditional adversarial positioning of medicine vs. administration is being consciously challenged and new roles and activities are being invented and designed that foster collaboration and cooperation. This new "partnership" may be the key to future viability, and many professional resources are being focused on the development of methods to assist in accomplishing this goal. The active involvement of the physician-manager may be the single most critical element in this process.

The first step is to strengthen the formal medical staff organization. Bylaws must be reviewed in light of current impacts from external sources, medical staff leadership must be enhanced and developed, and active participation in the organization by all members must be encouraged.

The next step is to provide training and education for the development of leadership and managerial skills of the medical staff, and then to provide structured opportunities for actual integration with management staff through team and group development activities. Each group expresses unique characteristics and cherishes certain values and self-images that are usually misperceived and misunderstood by the other. This results in negative and adversarial perceptions and attitudes.

Upon examination, the two groups actually share many values, expectations, and goals, but there are major differences in how they are communicated and what methods are developed for their achievement. The development of a common language, a clearer communication system, joint planning and problem-solving activities, and joint education and training must be given priority if an integration effort is to be successful.

My experience and data strongly suggest that all health care organizations, from single specialty groups to large comprehensive medical centers, need to first initiate an objective organizational assessment and analysis process to determine their current situation and state of integration. Second, a process of mutual goal setting and strategic planning must be established. Third, an integrated effort for planning and initiating activities that will lead to the desired change and/or objective must be developed.

An honest commitment to the development of collaboration and integration efforts by all parties may well be the key to future survival and viability. Assisting health care organizations in meeting this commitment is one of the primary roles and responsibilities of the physician executive and may be the most successful way to reduce the conflict and frustration of the dual role dilemma.

Part **II**

The Emerging Role

Commentary

The Physician Executive: Human Being, Manager, and Juggler

Don E. Detmer, M.D.

The physician executive has an important and inherently challenging role in the American health care environment. As both doctor and director, the physician executive straddles two domains—clinical medicine and organizational management—and must balance and integrate the concerns, knowledge, and skills of each. These two domains, medicine and management, are highly dynamic, responding to social, political, technologic, and economic developments, and will remain so into the new century. This means that change and opportunities for leadership are and will be integral parts of the physician executive's professional world and of the particular organization he or she helps direct. It is likely that the physician executive will be pivotal in developing and implementing health and social policy, as well as new clinical and organizational strategies, at the local level. Thus, the role holds unparalleled opportunity for leadership in medicine, management, and the larger community, leadership that can have significant implications for preserving health and reducing human suffering.

There are many books and articles about the management skills and attributes that are essential to executive success in general. Which of these faculties is most germane to the roles and responsibilities of the clinician executive? Of course, the physician executive shares many characteristics with executives in other fields. Like all executives, the physician executive is called upon to juggle successfully three areas of responsibility requiring different knowledge and skills. The first responsibility is defining the direction in which the institution (or group) is—or should be—headed. The organization's goals must be clarified, priorities set, and plans, timetables, strategies, and tactics generated to achieve them. The second responsibility is creating and maintaining the organizational structure and ensuring that all components work well in and of themselves so that as a group they promote the organization's goals. The third responsibility is managing people, which, in its broadest sense, includes communications, teaching, promoting employee productivity and growth, rewarding achievement, and dealing with conflicts within the organization. Good personnel management ensures that the organization's work gets done well and that the organization, like its team members, thrives.

Like any other manager, the physician executive also needs to have good instincts about organizational behavior. Knowing how to work within the organizational system and having an intuitive feel for the organization's ability to tolerate and adjust to change and challenge are important qualifications for any successful executive, as is having the instinct for knowing when to make, share, or delay decisions. Organizations have different needs at different times: the executive must be alert to signals from inside and outside the organization that may herald changing needs and indicate an urgency for new managerial responses. Indeed, because of his or her medical training, the physician executive may find it easier than will most other executives to see and understand the organization as a system of complex human social behavior or as an organic system with functional needs and a life all its own. On the other hand, to work well within the group dynamics of the organization and to find common ground for organizational planning, the physician executive must learn to temper clinical medicine's traditional insistence on physician autonomy, its assumption of the physician prerogative, and its absolute perseveration in individual cases. This means that one must be prepared and willing to engage physician colleagues who hold to the view that each doctor is a court unto himself or herself, and who will bristle at "group think" or "bureaucratese" and resist any and all efforts toward cooperative attainment of organizational goals. These skills are critical if one is to be more than just a simple caretaker of a highly complex enterprise.

How does the role of the clinician executive differ from that of other executives? What skills do physician executives need that other managers may not? These are key questions. The crucial differences between many social service, business, and industrial enterprises and the enterprise of contemporary health care seem to relate to the technology and traditions of health care. The physician executive needs not only the skills and attributes typically required of any executive but also special expertise to manage the powerful technologies, the dominant professional personalities (in great numbers), and the special human needs involved in health care. The task is to match these critical resources—technology and a professional labor force—with the particular health needs of the community to create a system able to improve the health of all citizens.

Health care technology today is a potent combination of highly specialized strategies, sophisticated and costly equipment, and individualized decision making (for example, deciding who needs coronary artery bypass surgery as opposed to balloon dilatation or medication). Both the technology and the knowledge needed to drive these decisions require highly developed skills. Without doubt, the physician executive plays and will continue to play a central role in the use, control, diffusion, and assessment of health care technology. He or she must become (and remain) familiar with emerging technologies and their applications as well as with the "bigger picture" of health care.

As we move toward the twenty-first century, there will be continuing pressure on the health care industry from outside to define value in health care as a blend of professional and traditional consumer expectations and assessments. There will be pressure, too, probably escalating pressure, to achieve significant cost savings. Health care will be expected to become more productive and to adjust its environment and practices to promote achievement of equal or better outcomes using equal or fewer resources. We are on the threshold of making clinical medicine far more scientific and accountable through application of the information sciences. This will require, among other things, more sophisticated computerized data systems and more intense real-time management of personnel and supplies. It will also place a greater premium on the quality of the interaction of the health professionals, administrative personnel, and public and corporate officials who comprise the management team.

The nature of the collective personalities of the health professions may well require special management consideration. The physician executive's colleagues and co-workers include many health professionals, including physicians, nurses, dentists, psychologists, and various allied health personnel. Each professional subgroup has its own tradition, perspective, role definition, and self-image; each requires special consideration as it is brought into alignment with other professional groups in the organization. For example, as mentioned above, physicians' traditional understanding of their autonomy in clinical medicine can pose significant problems for organizational management and for the manager. Although medicine and, consequently, the role of the physician have changed dramatically in the past 25 years, enough of the old view of physician autonomy remains among doctors today and is operative in their behavior that the clinician executive will be neither effective nor long in the job if he or she fails to recognize and accommodate this management reality. The physician executive must hold a broader perspective on issues of both clinical care and corporate management, one that takes account of and does not denigrate the particular views and contributions of various health care specialties. Maintaining credibility with and confidence in doctors and other practitioners "in the trenches" is essential to the success of the clinician executive, particularly in a changing health care environment. Achieving this is not easy, however, and requires ongoing education, clear communication, and boundless energy and enthusiasm.

Human needs at the heart of the health care enterprise call for a particular sensitivity in the management of health care organizations that may not be required in other corporate settings. The physician executive must demonstrate a feel for and knowledge of health and disease, diagnosis and treatment, and costs and benefits. He or she must also champion a commitment to human and social issues in health care. In addition to responding to patients' needs for clinical evaluation and treatment, good health care is reflective of the interrelatedness of health problems and social conditions, the values and ethics of health care, and the fact that the illness experience holds special meaning for patients. For example, comprehensive care for persons with acquired immunodeficiency syndrome (AIDS) entails not only good medical treatment of disease but sensitivity to patients' preferences and legal rights, integrated hospital and community-based care, preventive health education in the community, and even social interventions intended to give young people sufficient skills and self-assurance to avoid drug use and sexual behaviors that are linked epidemiologically to AIDS. Management decision makers in health care organizations must give consideration to the human and social dimensions of health care. The physician executive can sustain and reinforce the humanistic conscience of the organization, thereby balancing its entrepreneurial concerns with a dedication to human health and well-being.

There are two types of physician executives. The first is an individual who possesses a medical degree but who sees himself or herself primarily as a manager working at some real and/or psychological distance from the practice setting. The second is an individual who is clinically active but is also working as a leader in the interface between full-time clinicians and full-time administrators. The cases that follow depict physician executives of both types. By studying these cases, colleagues may gain a better understanding of the expectations and tensions unique to each type.

In his work on occupational socialization, E. H. Schein describes three types of managers: custodians, content innovators, and role innovators. Custodians, as might be expected, are managers who work within and seek to maintain established professional norms and current knowledge and technology bases. Content innovators accept traditional performance norms but seek to advance and change the knowledge base and technology of their field. Role innovators seek to redefine the respective roles and performance standards of the principals (manager, employee, practitioner, client, consumer, patient, and so on) in a professional enterprise. In so doing they may also redefine the scope and boundaries of the entire enterprise. Role innovators, says Schein, have as a chief concern making their professions more responsive to pressing social realities.[1]

All three types of physician executives are at work today in the U.S. health care system. But what the United States will need most in coming years are physician executives who are, in Schein's terms, innovators, both of content and of role. These innovators will have to possess the considerable skills required to define, implement, and manage constructive change in the health care system. They will have to take on, in active managerial decision making at the local level, the thorniest problems of American health care—quality, financing, and access.

Of all medical specialists, physician executives face perhaps the greatest challenges and opportunities. To practice "executive medicine" with competence and grace in the years just ahead presents a challenge more formidable than that of achieving distinction in any given clinical specialty. This is perhaps the best justification for making the physician executive's role explicit in the domains of professional education, management, practice, and public service.

The Part II Cases

In the four cases that follow the physician executives face various problems: unnecessary surgery, priorities for capital equipment, time prioritizing for a busy medical director, and clinical staffing at a nursing home. These problems are not simple. They may be symptoms of deeper conflicts between boards, management, and physicians over whom an organization serves and should serve, and in what ways and at what cost. The cases raise questions about how physician executives reconcile accountability to their employer organization and to the physicians they "manage."

Dr. Silver and unnecessary surgery

Dr. Silver takes seriously his job as chair of the obstetrics-gynecology department. He must be doing an acceptable job, or he wouldn't have been re-elected to his second five-year term. When he is presented with information by the hospital's surgical review committee that suggests that unnecessary surgery is being performed, he feels obligated to investigate the issue. He discovers that the alleged unnecessary surgery is being performed by two doctors in the same practice who supervise the residency training at the Medicaid clinic. He asks the physicians to present the cases at the monthly department meetings. He finds out that the cases were "grudgingly" accepted. When the same pattern continues, Dr. Silver suggests to the hospital's medical board that the physicians be supervised. The board is concerned about a lawsuit and so backs off the case.

As a physician executive, Dr. Silver has a responsibility to manage his department. This means supervising his personnel and at the same time making sure that high-quality care is provided to all patients being serviced by his department. There is a hint that some of the alleged unnecessary surgery is being performed on poor women. The ethical implications are numerous.

The suggestion is made that questioning the practices of the two physicians will threaten the reputation of the hospital and result in the expense of a lawsuit. Just how far should Dr. Silver stick his neck out?

Case questions

1. What is the problem?
2. What are the causes of the problem?
3. What are the options available to Dr. Silver?
4. What are the implications of each option?
5. What do you recommend?
6. Discuss the constraints and opportunities Dr. Silver faces in implementing your recommendations.

Northeast Medical Center

Northeast Medical Center is caught up in the postmerger blues. The medical staff wanted all inpatient facilities to be located at West Campus, but because of financial constraints and public pressure, the services were referred to East Campus, downtown. As a result of the controversy, relationships between administration and the medical staff have deteriorated.

The physician executive in this case, Dr. Arnold Schwartz, must possess a keen understanding of organizational behavior. This understanding must be balanced by his knowledge of sound financial management. At issue is the capital expenditure for two modern cystoscopy tables. The urologists seem to think the decision to place the new tables at West Campus was a bad one. They intend to flex their muscles and take their patients elsewhere.

Is the cystoscopy table the real issue, or are the dynamics between power groups really the problem?

Case questions

1. What are the facts of the case?
2. What would constitute a win/win solution for Dr. Schwartz, Chief of Urology, and Mr. Muldoon, President and CEO?
3. What options are available to Dr. Schwartz?
4. What are the implications of each option?
5. What do you recommend and why?
6. What are the opportunities and constraints Dr. Schwartz faces in implementing your recommendations?

Medical director in-basket exercise

Time management is a necessary survival skill for all successful executives. Crises happen, even to organized managers, and consequently, other activities are postponed. Problems pile up, secretaries take vacations, and Monday morning usually rolls around too quickly.

Time cannot be managed until the difference between how time is being used and how it should be used is understood. This distinction can be clarified by actually logging activities to find out how much time is being spent, where it is being spent, and why it is being spent. This will also illustrate the usefulness of setting priorities. Priority setting is a dynamic process of anticipating problems before they arise and responding to problems when they do arise. A manager must understand which priorities have already been set, the number of people affected by the alternative solutions, and the purpose and consequences of each alternative. Priority setting is a wasted effort unless resources are committed toward achieving the highest priority.

Being a good manager also means delegating responsibility. Which decisions can be made by someone else? To what extent are employees encouraged to make decisions without approval? How well are support staff utilized?

Procrastinators have special sets of problems and sometimes need help in modifying their behavior (for example, establishing personal penalties or rewards). Some mangers find it helpful to create written reminders and make lists. Taking one task at a time, finishing it, and bringing it to closure helps prevent scattered energy. When going through an in-basket, being realistic about what can be accomplished and when it can be accomplished will not only save time, it will also reduce stress.

Case questions

1. For each item in the in-basket, indicate a priority (emergent, urgent, routine), action necessary, and who is responsible.
2. For each problem area, list reasons why the problem occurred.
3. What are the options available to Dr. Olson in limiting the demands on her time?
4. What do you recommend and why?
5. Discuss the constraints and opportunities Dr. Olson faces in implementing your recommendations.

Medical care delivery at Saint Augustine Nursing Home

Sometimes it is too easy to forget the elderly residing in nursing homes. Because the population of the United States is quickly becoming an aged one, more attention is being devoted to the specialty of geriatric medicine.

Mr. Williams, Saint Augustine's administrator, was hired because of his progressive approach to the nursing home industry. Mr. Williams, in turn, hired the progressive Dr. Michaels as the new half-time medical director. Mr. Williams was looking for a physician executive who had formal geriatric training and who would make sure that good care was being provided to every nursing home resident.

The system, however, was entrenched in the medical care model that allowed each resident to choose and use their personal physician. Both Mr. Williams and Dr. Michaels believed that this model led to a lower standard of care than the patients rightfully could receive. What kind of model is best? How should it be changed?

Case questions

1. What is the problem?
2. What is the cause of the problem?
3. What are the options available to Dr. Michaels?
4. Which options is Dr. Michaels likely to recommend?
5. Do you agree with Dr. Michaels's recommendations and why? If you do not agree, why do you differ from Dr. Michaels?
6. What are the opportunities and constraints Dr. Michaels faces in implementing his or your recommendations?

Note

1. E. H. Schein, *Organizational Psychology*, 2d ed. (Englewood Cliffs, NJ: Prentice Hall, 1970).

Case 1

Dr. Silver and Unnecessary Surgery

Abraham M. Lenobel, M.D.

Atlantic Hospital is a 430-bed community hospital in the northeast sector of the United States. It is a suburban hospital that serves an area with a base population of about 300,000 people. There is an active obstetric-gynecology (OB-GYN) department with 25 members. Approximately 2,300 deliveries, 720 major gynecologic procedures, and more than 1,100 minor procedures are done each year. As one might expect, the distribution of cases among the staff is not equal. Several groups do more work, proportionally, and several individuals and groups do much less. The OB-GYN staff is divided into two groups of four-person practices, three groups of three-person practices, three groups of two-person practices, and two solo practitioners. There is a fairly large Medicaid clinic supervised by one of the three-person groups of attendings on the staff at the hospital. The hospital also provides a training setting for general practice residents from a nearby school of medicine that has an approved residency and also uses the facilities of several hospitals in the community for training in various specialties.

Richard Silver, M.D., is the chair of the department of obstetrics and gynecology. He is in his mid-50s and has been practicing in the community for 22 years. He is a member of one of the three-person practices. Silver is in his seventh year as the chair of the department, having been reelected by the department to a second five-year term. As the head of a clinical department in the hospital, he is a voting member of the hospital's medical board.

About 15 months ago, the surgical review committee forwarded to Dr. Silver several cases, which had been collected over previous months, that had postoperative diagnoses that did not conform to the preoperative diagnoses. There were several cases of hysterectomy for fibroids. On some charts the preoperative examination documented enlarged uteri some eight to ten weeks in gestational size, but the pathology examination reported uteri weighing 100 to 130 grams, that is, well within the average weights of a normal uterus. Some pathology reports did not confirm the presence of fibroids, and some pathology reports documented fibroids so small that they did not enlarge the uterus. Each of these cases was reviewed by Dr. Silver and presented at the monthly clinical department meetings. At these meetings the two gynecologists who performed the surgeries provided additional information. The treatment in the cases was grudgingly accepted by the department as "borderline" justified.

The utilization review committee reported cases of women with menorrhagia (heavy menstrual bleeding) who were admitted for hysterectomies by the same two gynecologists. Menorrhagia may or may not cause low blood counts, depending on treatment, and might be considered an indication for hysterectomy, if a low blood count or anemia is present. Anemia must be persistent or recurrent in spite of treatment to justify a hysterectomy. These patients' hemoglobin levels were within normal range and no anemia was documented. The cases were reviewed retrospectively and were also brought to the department monthly meetings for discussion. The committee also found and reported that a disproportionate number of cases were admitted by the two gynecologists for exploratory laporatomy with a diagnosis of infertility. The operative notes for these cases reported "lysis of adhesions" as the main surgical procedure.

The cases were difficult to justify. Dr. Silver again put the cases on the agenda for the department meeting and personally discussed the cases with the two gynecologists under consideration. He believed that their performance represented a persistent pattern of unjustified surgery. Since the pattern had not changed, even after review and meetings, he brought the problem to the medical board. The medical board discussed the problem but could not agree with Dr. Silver's request to place the two gynecologists on supervision. They feared that it would be an invitation to legal action and would reflect poorly on the medical staff and the hospital.

The first gynecologist, Dr. Berley, was in his early 60s and had been practicing in the area for 26 years. He received his undergraduate medical education overseas, and interned and did residency training in an acceptable program. The second gynecologist, Dr. West, was in his late 40s and had been associated with Dr. Berley for 17 years. He trained in a prestigious northeastern medical school and did his residency training in an outstanding university hospital. The third member of their group had been with the group for five years and received undergraduate training in an acceptable program in the mid-Atlantic states. The third gynecologist was only involved in the surgical cases in question by providing assistance at surgery, and only had an occasional case reported to the Chair by one of the quality review committees.

This three-person group supervised the residency training program that staffed the Medicaid clinic, and several of the cases under consideration involved Medicaid patients. One of the solo practitioners in the area had been associated with the two gynecologists in this three-person group, but for reasons that were unknown, he broke away from the partnership arrangement and established his own practice in the same community. His work was never under question.

Dr. Silver made an appointment with one of the assistant hospital administrators and presented the above situation to him. The assistant administrator advised a conference with the administrator and legal counsel prior to any action. This meeting was arranged for the following month. Dr. Silver, Mr. Robbins (the senior administrator of the hospital), and Mr. Lee, a representative of a legal firm on retainer to the hospital as counsel, were present at the meeting. Dr. Silver reported the sequence of events and a lively discussion took place.

Several points were brought up for consideration. Dr. Silver was advised that although he served in an administrative capacity on a voluntary unremunerated basis, in reality he could be considered to be in competition with the physicians under consideration because his professional group was in direct competition with the professional group whose members were under discussion. Dr. Silver was also informed that his malpractice insurer, which was the carrier for the hospital as well, would cover malpractice insurance. Unfortunately, it would not provide coverage for any suit that might be brought against him for harassment or malicious mischief. If the two physicians under consideration by Dr. Silver were placed under either supervisory or restrictive limitations, they in turn might institute legal proceedings against both the hospital and Dr. Silver personally as director of the department. Mr. Robbins, representing the hospital, was hesitant to return to the medical board to request restrictive measures, especially in view of the fact that the three-person group under consideration had no admitting or surgical privileges at any other hospital in the area. Mr. Robbins also pointed out that he had discussed the situation with members of the hospital's board of directors. If suits were brought for malicious mischief or harassment, the hospital's malpractice carrier would not cover the defense, nor would the hospital be covered by any other insurance. The hospital would be forced to pay for its (and possibly Dr. Silver's) defense out of hospital funds. These costs might not be included under some of the third party reimbursement calculations. Therefore, the hospital would have to pay these legal fees. Mr. Robbins intimated that the board would prefer to retain the status quo.

Dr. Silver left the meeting in considerable distress. He had information that indicated that excessive and unnecessary surgery was being performed and that unneeded medical care was being rendered. He was also concerned that this type of care might be learned by the residents. His intervention would put him into possible personal jeopardy, and he would not be insured and might not have coverage for legal defense by either the hospital or his own carrier. Should a suit ensue from any corrective measures he would think indicated, he might ultimately have to undertake his own defense. Measures he had taken to bring the problems to departmental notice had not achieved a change in the behavior patterns of the physicians. The medical board was not helpful. He was not being backed by the hospital's administration. Dr. Silver did not know which way to turn.

Northeast Medical Center

Howard E. Rotner, M.D.

Dr. Arnold Schwartz, Medical Director of Northeast Medical Center, opened his mail on 14 September to find a copy of a letter sent by Dr. David Kinder, Chief of the Department of Urology, to the other chiefs of staff. The letter read as follows:

Dear Chiefs of Staff:

You have rightfully come to expect a high degree of expertise and technology from the urology service in our hospitals. There are going to be dramatic changes from what you have come to expect starting on October 15th. After October 15th, we (Urology) will be faced with having inpatients in a hospital with an antiquated cystoscopy table and no provisions for outpatients. On the other hand, the best cystoscopy table north of the city will be located in the former West Hospital—an ambulatory care center with no ICU, no laboratory, no x-ray, and no nighttime house staff. This table is needed for all modern urologic endoscopic procedures.

Many sick patients may have to be taken care of in a facility other than Northeast so that potential risks can be avoided. Hopefully, you will be understanding of our situation. We will try not to inconvenience you or your patients. I am sure you will agree that quality of care for the patients is of the utmost importance. This situation will not change until Northeast Medical Center can find the funds to switch the two cysto tables. We need your help.

David Kinder, M.D.
Chief, Department of Urology

The Medical Center

Northeast Medical Center is a 354-bed, not-for-profit community hospital located in a town approximately ten miles north of a large city. The medical center is located on two campuses—East Campus and West Campus—and was formed when two separate not-for-profit community hospitals, with a total of 501 beds, merged into one entity. The merger occurred over a period of approximately five years. Northeast Medical Center now has one board of trustees, one chief executive officer (CEO), and one medical staff under one set of bylaws. As a result of the merger, all acute care medical/surgical and obstetrical beds are located at East Campus. Outpatient activities, including the surgicenter, a walk-in center, and a 24-bed inpatient mental health unit, are located at West Campus. As a result of the merger, 147 beds were eliminated from the two hospitals.

The merger has taken its toll upon each of the two hospitals, individually as well as collectively. Considerable controversy was attached to the merger because the town council, the majority of the town's inhabitants and their advocacy groups, and the local health planning council all wanted the inpatient beds to remain at East Campus. The medical staff, on the other hand, preferred to locate the inpatient beds at West Campus with an expansion of that campus to accommodate approximately 150 more beds. The proposal was opposed by the various neighborhood groups at each campus, and eventually financial constraints became so severe that the only available alternative for the medical center was to utilize the East Campus facility as the major inpatient acute care facility.

The controversy caused moderate attrition of the medical staff to other competing hospitals in nearby towns. The medical staff also has given the chief executive officer, Mr. Muldoon, two unanimous votes of "no confidence" during the past year. The medical center is trying desperately to maintain its market share in order to preserve its volume, and it realizes that the loyalty of the medical staff is critical to this end.

The Administration of Northeast Medical Center

Mr. Timothy Muldoon has been the president and chief executive officer of Northeast Medical Center for the past three years. Mr. Muldoon, a former executive at a local bank and member of the board of trustees of the former East Campus hospital, assumed the position of president and CEO of the medical center after several previous administrators resigned. Mr. Muldoon is a highly intelligent man who is authoritative and autocratic in his management style. He has worked hard to develop good relations with physicians and has supported joint ventures with many members of the medical staff. Nevertheless, he has little experience in health care and, in the eyes of the medical staff, has a poor understanding of physician behavior. He invariably sees physician behavior as immature, impulsive, and detrimental to the goals of the medical center. In an environment of staff reduction, cost cutting, and fiscal restraint, Mr. Muldoon is viewed by the medical staff as the individual responsible for the sacrifice of high-quality care in order to cut costs.

Arnold Schwartz has been the medical director of Northeast Medical Center since September of 1985. For the previous 17 years, he was a practicing internist and endocrinologist with a large and strong internal medicine group. Dr. Schwartz has had to walk a fine line between the medical staff and the administration during the extremely controversial period of the merger and other cost-cutting measures. He has managed this task very well and is held in high esteem by both the medical staff and the administration. While he is considered an individual of high integrity and fairness, there are still many members of the medical staff who are suspicious of his role and would not hesitate to attack him should they feel that he has become a tool of the administration. Dr. Schwartz sometimes is viewed as compromising quality by the medical staff in their battle against cost and staff reductions. His failure to deliver on issues of quality is perceived by the medical staff as failing to perform his duty as the guardian of high-quality care.

Cathleen O'Brien is Director of Marketing and Planning at Northeast Medical Center. She has been with the medical center for approximately three years. She is an experienced health care professional who started as a registered nurse and ultimately rose through the ranks and obtained a master's degree in business administration. She has worked for for-profit companies and is perceived as having a "for-profit viewpoint." She is an individual capable of producing a prodigious amount of work, and Mr. Muldoon relies heavily on her opinions. Her duties during the consolidation and merger process have included responsibility for all of the facility planning and renovations. She is responsible for the cystoscopy room renovations and the exchange of cystoscopy tables that would allow the inpatient facility at East Campus to have the state-of-the-art equipment. Ms. O'Brien is perceived as a driven individual who, because of her close relationship with Mr. Muldoon, retains an enormous amount of power in the medical center. She has poor communications with other members of administration and the medical staff, who have accused her of withholding information for manipulative purposes. Although she is not well liked by many people in the medical center, she nevertheless commands a good deal of respect for her knowledge, commitment, and capabilities.

Dr. David Kinder is Chief of the Department of Urology. He is a 42-year-old physician who is energetic, outspoken, and highly regarded for his surgical skills. Dr. Kinder's methods of expression exemplify, in Mr. Muldoon's eyes, the type of behavior that is detrimental to the ultimate goals of the medical center. Mr. Muldoon feels that Dr. Kinder is using his power unfairly by uniting the other service chiefs behind his goals and not rationally discussing the situation in a less explosive environment. To make matters worse, Dr. Kinder is the younger associate of Dr. John Boccio, the past president of the medical staff, who led the no-confidence votes against Mr. Muldoon. Mr. Muldoon suspects there is some element of conspiracy behind the ostensible issue of updating the cystoscopy table at East Campus. He wonders how to address the faction forming within the staff in a way that will bring about more constructive relationships and unified goals.

Medical Director In-Basket Exercise: Time Management at the O. P. Melius Medical Center

Jeffrey Kunz, M.D.

"Late again!" muttered Ingrid K. Olson, M.D., as she quickly parked her car at 8:00 on a Monday morning in the rain-soaked physicians' parking lot. These days the 45-year-old medical director of the O. P. Melius Medical Center never seemed to have enough time. Several months into her job, she now realized that serving as the chief medical officer of a 100-plus physician multispecialty group was not exactly the "piece of cake" that she thought it to be during her years of active practice and research.

Dr. Olson had returned Saturday night from a 10-day residential session for clinician executives at the University of Wisconsin in Madison. She enjoyed these on-campus segments of her two-year postgraduate program and felt better prepared to handle the demands of the job, which she assumed after the sudden death of the former medical director.

Still, she would be glad to get her master's degree in administrative medicine next spring so she would have more time for her work, family, and recreation—not necessarily in that order!

She realized that she faced a tough week ahead. Besides the backlog of work undoubtedly waiting on her desk, she had to put the finishing touches on a cost-containment speech she was to give at noon to the Downtown Rotary Club, and find time to complete an assignment to be discussed tomorrow night on the weekly teleconference session for one of her graduate courses.

"It could be worse," she thought to herself. Since her long-time secretary, Phyllis Ribbons, also was returning to work that day from a week-long vacation/sales convention with her husband in Hawaii, Dr. Olson had scheduled a lighter than usual day to enable both of them to catch up.

On the way to her office, she stopped by the cafeteria to get her obligatory morning cup of coffee and was delighted to see her secretary a few steps ahead. This morning, however, Phyllis looked tired and a bit frazzled standing in line and fidgeting with her change purse.

"Welcome back, Phyllis. Is that Kona coffee in your cup?" teased Dr. Olson.

"I only wish it were Ingrid," replied Phyllis softly. "We had plane and weather troubles connecting in San Francisco, and I've just come from the airport. After a quick peek at your office and what is waiting, I'm not sure that either of us will be glad to be back!"

After paying for the coffee, the two hurriedly exited the cafeteria, and Ms. Ribbons related to Dr. Olson some of the problems that she had discovered on arriving 15 minutes earlier.

The conference room where Dr. Olson was to hold her usual Monday morning management meeting with her division and department heads in less than an hour had been flooded during heavy rains over the weekend. Water damage had also knocked out, hopefully only temporarily, their office voice-mail system, so only a large pile of written telephone messages, mail, memos, and fax messages were immediately available for Dr. Olson's review.

Phyllis explained apologetically that the secretary covering for her had scheduled a number of meetings today for Dr. Olson after checking with Rod Kaiser. Mr. Kaiser was the administrator and chief operating officer of the medical center and had agreed to cover for Dr. Olson only after she assured him that he would be in charge during her absence. Both Dr. Olson and Mr. Kaiser reported to the CEO, Dr. Koshgarian.

Dr. Olson sat at her desk, reviewed the following schedule and messages, and began to set priorities for the day and the week. She wondered if the job needed to be this stressful or if changes in the medical center were indicated.

Item 1: Schedule

Scheduled Appointments for Ingrid Olson, M.D.
Monday, June 3

  8:30   Clinical directors meeting

9:00   Clinical directors meeting

9:30   Return telephone calls

10:00   Paul Sobicinski

10:30   Bea Cho, M.D., Ph.D.

11:00   Return telephone calls

11:30   Leave for Downtown Rotary Club (DRC) at the Riverside Club

12:00   DRC fundraising speech for children's unit

12:30   "   "   "   "   "   "

1:00   "   "   "   "   "   "

1:30   Return telephone calls

2:00   open

2:30   open

3:00   Alfred Epstein, M.D.

3:30   Julia Whitehorse, R.N.

4:00   Rod Kaiser (his office)

4:30   Return telephone calls

6:00   Nellie's open house (Theodore Roosevelt Elementary)

7:00   Medical Staff Executive Committee (MD dining room)

Item 2: FAX message

TO: Ingrid K. Olson, M.D.
             Administration
FROM: Daniel R. Hammer, M.D., F.A.C.S.
             Orthopaedic Surgery
DATE: June 3
SUBJECT: Surgical Outreach

Just to brighten your day, I want to share some good news! A surgical colleague of mine asked if I would travel on Wednesdays (my day off) to his community to do consultations and perhaps some surgery.

Seeing this as a win/win, I tentatively said yes. I could use the extra money and the area could benefit from my skills. Do you see any problems with this? I would like to start Wednesday, June 5.

Item 3: Telephone message, Thursday, May 30

Gwen Garcia, Provider Relations Coordinator of Preferred Physicians Health Plan, called to discuss contracting for medical services. Please call on Monday, June 3, between 9 and 11 A.M.

Item 4: Memo

TO: Dr. Ingrid Olson, Medical
FROM: Hank Best, Management Services
DATE: May 29
SUBJECT: Parking Problems

We continue to have problems with medical staff who park in the doctors' lot without permits affixed to their left rear window. Also, some are asking for more than the two stickers allocated to each medical staff member!

Effective next week, we will tow any vehicle parked in our designated doctors' lot not displaying a valid permit.

cc: Mr. Rod Kaiser

Item 5: Electronic mail message (22:53:17 hrs 29 May)

Dear Ingrid:

Heard that you have been busy as a bee in the spring, but what gives? You promised me with uncrossed fingers and no hands behind your back that you would have your chapter for our book in my hot hands by 15 April.

Please e-mail or fax reply stat. Better yet, send manuscript draft by overnight courier to the publisher.

Fretfully yours,

David Goodfriend

Item 6: Letter, May 18

Dear Dr. Olson:

I am writing to thank you and your staff for the high quality and kind care that my father, James L. Jones, received from the medical team led by Dr. Ralph Gunnar.

Dad died last month at home after a long illness made so much more tolerable by your physicians, nurses, and home health aides. Enclosed are checks given in lieu of flowers by his American Legion buddies, church, and family members.

We wish it could be more, for we know that you will put it to good use. God bless you all.

Sincerely,

Aurelia Jones Tyler
(Mrs. T. H.)

P.S. Please contact me if you need any more volunteers at the medical center.

Item 7: Urgent attention slip, June 1

ATTN: Ingrid Olson, M.D.
O. P. Melius Medical Center

Would you please sign the attached grant applications and cover sheets on the lines indicated? They have all passed our institutional review board and in-house peer review.

Please have Phyllis call me as soon as you are done so I can send them to Washington by express mail. Sorry for this last minute request, but we have been working on them literally day and night.

When you get a free moment, please give me a call to follow up on last month's discussion of additional research space.

Thanks,

Felix Wu, Ph.D.

Item 8: Telephone message, June 3

Philip Patel of Guardian News Service called to "confirm some facts on a story about to break." Please call him by 10 A.M. today at the latest.

Item 9: Letter, May 16

Dear Doctor Olson:

Anna B. Turkevich, M.D., a former employee of your organization has applied for membership in our county medical society. At your earliest convenience would you please give us your frank assessment of Doctor Turkevich's professional ability, personal character, and ethical demeanor? Attached is a signed release from the applicant.

Thanking you in advance, I remain

Very truly yours,

F. L. Lounsberry, M.D., F.A.C.P.
Secretary

Item 10: Telephone message, June 3

Dr. Koshgarian called on his way to the airport and asked that you call him back on his mobile phone before 9 A.M. or at his daughter's home in Bethesda tonight after 7 P.M.

Item 11: Memo

CONFIDENTIAL MEMORANDUM

TO:	Ingrid K. Olson, M.D.
	Chief Medical officer
FROM:	Alfred R. Epstein, M.D.
	Chief of Radiology
DATE:	May 31
SUBJECT:	Resignation

It is with sincere regret and much frustration that I submit this letter of resignation. I am sorry to send this to you while you are out of town as I have valued our friendship since your student days. Considered calling you in Wisconsin but decided to discuss it with you after I cool down and you get back to the medical center.

Never in 34 years of practice have I seen the kind of bureaucratic interference that has plagued my department these past two weeks. Please have Phyllis obtain the necessary papers, including my pension and profit-sharing termination notice. I do not have the strength to have my staff or myself go another round in the ring.

Ingrid, better get your own golden parachute ready. These guys do not play by the rules!

Item 12: Memo

TO:	Ingrid Olson, M.D.
	Medical Director
FROM:	Dorothy Bergmann, M.D., M.P.H.
	Director of Medical Education
DATE:	May 24
SUBJECT:	Lecture to First-Year Residents

Enjoyed your recent grand rounds presentation on continuous quality improvement. Would you be willing to do it again on Wednesday, June 26, at 10 A.M. for new resident orientation?

Have a good trip to the Badger State.

Item 13: Letter, May 22

Dear Dr. Olson:

On my morning walks I notice that when the medical center has its trash picked up, red-bagged infectious waste is being put out along with the usual trash and recyclables. You probably do not realize that this is happening, but as a neighbor and fellow health professional I know this is not proper. Please correct this!

Sincerely,

A Concerned Neighbor

Item 14: Telephone message, May 24

Dr. Scopman called. He sees no reason why he should not put through full charges to our billing staff for "no show" patients. Will continue to do so unless he hears from you.

Item 15: Telephone message, May 30

Bunny Jones (Mrs. Thomas P.) wants to know the results of her husband's HIV testing. Has called three times as well as several calls to the laboratory and her husband's physician. Says she "can't get any answers." Referred to you by a friend.

Paul Sobicinski (Mrs. Jones' attorney) called twice. Also to Mr. Kaiser. Please return Mr. Sobicinski's call ASAP!

Item 16: Telephone message, May 31

Frank Mohammed, board member of Downtown Rotary, called to confirm arrangements for your Monday noon speech.

Also said that Dr. Koshgarian, "your boss," suggested he discuss with you the possibility of another Rotary member making a substantial donation to the children's treatment unit fund. Please return his call.

Item 17: Telephone message, June 3

Phil Gonzalez, owner of Precision Tool & Die, is angry that his employee, Frank Novak, is "getting the run-around" from our occupational health department. Wants an immediate response. "Can he return to work or not!"

Tried calling occupational health myself but no answer yet.

Item 18: Letter, May 22

Dear Doctor Olson:

You may remember at last month's medical center fashion fundraiser that I offered my professional services in interior design for the soon-to-be-renovated medical staff conference room in the south wing. My husband John, Chief of Vascular Surgery at your medical center, tells me that you are the person to contact.

Enclosed are completed designs for the conference room. I hope that you do not consider it presumptuous that I have gone ahead and done the plans, knowing that you will like them and that my fees are competitive.

Please call me upon your return to your office so that we may make any final revisions before you begin construction.

Cordially,

Helen Van Horn
Co-owner
Fin and Feather Design, Inc.

Item 19: Telephone message, May 31

Lisa Chaudwater from our Medicare intermediary called. Needs to set up a meeting with you to discuss some billing issues. Please return her call.

Item 20: Memo

CONFIDENTIAL MEMORANDUM

TO: Ingrid Olson, M.D.
           Medical Director & C.M.O.
FROM: Bea Cho, M.D.
           Department of Pathology
DATE: May 30
SUBJECT: Gross Negligence

I really need to talk with you about a quality-of-care issue concerning a physician colleague whom I believe is impaired. We had some problems last night that were unwarranted.

Please call me. We need to do something *now*.

Item 21: Telephone messages, May 31 and June 3

Dr. Cho called twice. Please call him as soon as you arrive.

Item 22: FAX message

TO: State Medical Society Committee on Tort Reform
FROM: John Alright, M.D., Chair
DATE: June 3
SUBJECT: Important Reception

I have just learned that State Senator and Majority Leader Chip Hale is having a reception (fundraiser) tonight at Boomer's Restaurant. I have been advised that a strong showing of our members tonight might persuade the senator to move our languishing bill along.

    Sorry for the short notice.

Item 23: Memo

TO: Ingrid Olson, M.D.
            Medical Director
FROM: Julia Whitehorse, M.S., R.N.
            Director of Nursing
DATE: May 29
RE: Possible air contamination

New telephone and air conditioning ducts are being installed in the ceiling space in the south wing. This apparently is causing white particles to fall down through the removed ceiling tiles into patient care areas. Several patients and staff have complained.

    Looking up into the ceiling space it looks like this white material comes from insulation sprayed on the steel support beams. I have discussed this problem with Hank Best, Director of Management Services, who says, "It's no big deal."

    I am concerned that we may be exposing people to asbestos. Would you please look into this or advise me how to proceed further? Thanks!

cc: Rod Kaiser, M.A.

Item 24: Telephone message, June 2

Please call ASAP Judy Netasinga, mother of pediatric patient Amy Netasinga. Needs to talk with you about an "important private matter."

Case 4

Medical Care Delivery at Saint Augustine Nursing Home

Barry M. Schultz, M.D.

Saint Augustine Nursing Home (SANH) is a 200-bed skilled nursing facility in Hometown, a small suburb in an East Coast metropolitan area. SANH recently applied successfully for a certificate of need to add 104 beds to the home. It is owned and operated by the Missionary Sisters, who also own and operate a 700-bed acute care hospital in the city. These institutions are nonprofit (voluntary). The sisters have a mission to provide the highest possible quality of care regardless of age, race, or ability to pay.

Mr. Williams, the home's administrator, was hired four years ago because of his progressive approach to the nursing home industry. His background in gerontological social work made him keenly sensitive to the special needs of the elderly in long-term care settings. After coming to SANH, Mr. Williams became concerned about the quality of medical care the residents received, but because of his lack of formal medical training he was unable to critically evaluate the quality of care. After due consideration, he gently encouraged the half-time medical director, Dr. Franklin, to retire. Although he was an octogenarian, Dr. Franklin did not have the background in geriatric medicine required to maintain a high quality of medical care.

When Dr. Franklin finally announced his retirement as medical director, Mr. Williams requested that the board of trustees approve the hiring of a new full-time medical director at a salary high enough to attract a physician with formal training in geriatrics. However, the board was concerned about the cost and did not want to spend too much money on a full-time medical director; the idea of the nursing home taking more responsibility for the quality of the medical care was not universally well received by the board members. They felt that quality-of-care issues should be left up to the individual residents' physicians.

The board did approve the hiring of a new half-time medical director at a slight increase over Dr. Franklin's salary, so Mr. Williams recruited a physician with formal training in geriatric medicine who was just finishing his geriatric fellowship training. Dr. Michaels was selected over several other more experienced candidates because of his formal geriatric training as well as his progressive approach to the care of the elderly. Mr. Williams hoped Dr. Michaels would corroborate his evaluation about the quality of medical care at SANH and would be able to find workable solutions to correct the deficiencies.

Soon after his arrival at SANH, Dr. Michaels concluded that the medical care at SANH was well below the standard he had seen in other nursing homes. He immediately began counseling the physicians delivering care at the home in an attempt to upgrade the quality of care. Unfortunately, he met with significant resistance among certain physicians when he suggested they change their approach to certain medical problems. These physicians were determined not to have their judgment questioned and resisted any attempts to be reeducated. It was hard to discipline the individual physicians because the formally organized medical staff at SANH protected its members.

Undaunted, Dr. Michaels began to develop a sophisticated quality assurance program designed to assess the content of care as well as compliance with documentation requirements. Mr. Williams fully supported and encouraged Dr. Michaels in his efforts. He assured the medical director that he would support his decision to remove any physician from the staff who did not comply with state guidelines for high-quality medical care.

Although there was a slight improvement in the quality of medical care, Dr. Michaels felt that the deficit that remained would be difficult to correct with the current approach. He believed that the basic problem originated in the medical care model being employed at SANH. Most of the residents at SANH received their medical care from one of six private physicians in the community who signed an agreement with the home. In addition to having active outpatient and acute care hospital private practices, each of these physicians provided all primary medical care services for a group of 25 to 30 residents of the home. The physicians received reimbursement directly from Medicare on a fee-for-service basis. This primary care group had a shared on-call system whereby each day one of the six physicians took calls for all of the primary care group's residents. Because SANH had a resident bill of rights that stated that any resident could be cared for by the physician of their choice, the remaining residents received primary care from their personal physicians. Physicians caring for individual residents ("courtesy staff") were responsible for providing their own 24-hour coverage.

Consultative care was provided by a group of specialist physicians who applied for privileges and were approved by a credentials committee made up of physicians on the medical staff and the medical director. When a resident required a consultation by a specialist, the resident's primary care physician requested a consultation from one of the approved physicians. All primary care physicians also had to be approved by the credentials committee. Consultants received reimbursement by billing Medicare.

Dr. Michaels was concerned that physicians in private practice were too busy to care adequately for the residents. Furthermore, most physicians had been trained to provide acute care, high-technology medicine. However, because the elderly tend to be frail, they do not tolerate procedure-oriented medicine well. In the geriatric populations that reside in nursing homes, some problems that need more attention are ignored because of lack of training or inattention on the part of the physicians. These problems require the type of multidisciplinary approach not normally included in traditional medical education. Medical schools have only recently begun teaching the principles of geriatric medicine that follow this approach.

In the first six months of his tenure as medical director, Dr. Michaels accumulated an impressive amount of anecdotal evidence pointing to suboptimal medical care. The evidence came from three areas: documentation, access, and style of practice.

In reviewing the charts of residents at Saint Augustine, Dr. Michaels found significant deficiencies in several aspects of medical documentation. For example, a significant number of monthly progress notes failed to include essential components, such as a medication list and a complete list of diagnoses. In addition, many notes did not reflect important events that had occurred during the previous month. A major gap in the medical records of many residents was a lack of documentation reflecting hospital transfers and readmissions. Finally, although good medical practice dictates that a progress note be written whenever a new condition or change in condition requires intervention, Dr. Michaels found many instances in which this had not been done.

With regard to access to care, Dr. Michaels found several disturbing examples in which residents had been denied prompt access to care because a physician was not available. Difficulty contacting physicians by telephone was a chronic problem that frequently required nursing staff to postpone critical interventions. In addition, there were instances in which physicians chose to give orders over the telephone when it would have been more appropriate to see the resident. There was also an occasional practice of inappropriately transferring the resident by ambulance to a local hospital emergency room for a simple examination. Even more disturbing was the evidence that certain physicians were spending little or no time with the resident when making a "visit."

As a formally trained geriatrician, Dr. Michaels had developed a style of practice that integrated medical issues with a person's social, psychological, and functional concerns. This framework usually resulted in medical decisions that departed significantly from those of physicians adhering to a more traditional medical model. As part of this somewhat different approach, the nature of care in a long-term care setting required each resident to have a practitioner willing to be their "case manager." The individual acting as the case manager needed to be familiar with all of the resident's particular needs and to address these in a multidisciplinary manner. Therefore, Dr. Michaels often became frustrated over what he considered the inappropriate medical care being delivered to the residents.

The delivery of long-term care is two-tiered because, although many of the needs of people residing in these facilities are custodial in nature, there are also many acute intermittent illnesses that require a more traditional type of medical intervention. The first tier, involving custodial care, requires the multidisciplinary approach rendered by a practitioner who can act as the case manager for the resident. The second tier, because it is acute and intermittent, more closely resembles traditional medical practice in that it involves the evaluation and treatment of diseases that are expected to have an endpoint. Because many aspects of long-term care cross over into both areas, the distinction between the two aspects of care is somewhat irrelevant. However, the division is helpful because it points out a major difference between traditional models of acute medical care and long-term care.

Dr. Michaels concluded that the medical care delivery model operating at SANH was not adequately meeting the needs of the residents at either of the two care levels. Although the physicians at SANH were not oriented toward the first level of care, these custodial services were provided by a well-structured multidisciplinary care team that reviewed residents' status and established goals for a set time period. Before Dr. Michaels arrived, the only discipline not represented on the team was medicine, and that was because the physicians were unable to take the time to be present for these meetings. Dr. Michaels attempted to circumvent this weakness in the multidisciplinary care team by representing the physicians at these meetings. He established a system of written communication so that he could make recommendations for modification of residents' care based on information obtained at these meetings.

Thus, residents were receiving adequate custodial care due to efforts of SANH staff, despite the physicians' lack of interest in this level of the two-tiered system of care. Still lacking was the concept of the case manager. Since the physicians did not accept the responsibility for this aspect of care, the role of the case manager was usually accepted by the head nurse on the nursing unit where the resident resided. Dr. Michaels did not find this inappropriate. The head nurse on each unit usually had a very good understanding of the resident's needs. His or her daily interaction with residents provided the global understanding necessary to assess various needs. The only problem with this system, as viewed by Dr. Michaels, was that, although it seemed to work well, it did not recognize (at least, officially) the critical role of the nurse as the case manager. It seemed to Dr. Michaels that nurses were not given an appropriate level of responsibility for making decisions regarding the resident's overall care. For example, when the head nurse became aware of a new problem that required a simple intervention, he or she had to call the physician to write an order for this intervention. The physician was then asked to make a decision about an issue that he or she knew very little about. Dr. Michaels concluded that many physicians in private practice were not prepared to deliver the custodial level of primary care required by these elderly residents.

The second level of the two-tiered care system was the care required by residents when they developed acute intermittent illnesses. In theory, it was the same type of care younger people living in the community received when they became ill. In the community setting, individuals who become ill contact their physician. In the long-term care situation, the nurse is usually the individual making contact with the physician on behalf of the resident. The physician must then make a special trip to the nursing home to render care. Dr. Michaels noticed that physicians were reluctant to make these special trips to the home. He speculated that the reasons might be that these trips took them away from their busy office and hospital practices, that they very well might not be reimbursed for these visits, and that certain "agist" attitudes among these physicians caused them to be less interested in providing needed care. Additionally, Dr. Michaels was concerned that these physicians were often making decisions for residents regarding the degree of care given, without first inquiring what the residents' preferences might be.

Dr. Michaels also discovered a disturbing habit about the way some of the physicians arranged to see residents who developed an acute intermittent illness. Instead of coming to the nursing home, these physicians would have the residents transferred to the emergency room of the local community hospital. This saved the physician from making a trip to the nursing home, since the physician was likely to be at the hospital for another reason. The physician was then able to charge for this type of visit, whereas he or she might not be able to do so for an intermittent visit to the nursing home. Dr. Michaels was concerned and felt this practice was a serious abuse of the system. In addition to causing the resident to undergo a very difficult ambulance transfer, it incurred a significant additional cost, without a comparable benefit, for the care the resident received.

This and other examples suggested that the physicians involved in delivering primary care at SANH were not well suited to handle either component of the two-tiered system. Dr. Michaels felt a different model of health care delivery would be required to correct these deficiencies. The concept of having physicians responsible for the primary care needs of nursing home residents was deeply rooted in the American medical tradition of each person having his or her own private physician. It is generally acknowledged that in the best medical care, physicians are present for all facets of the care. Dr. Michaels felt that the physicians delivering care at SANH were not rendering optimal care due to a combination of inadequate training as well as lack of attention to important issues.

When considering options for a new medical care delivery system, Dr. Michaels realized that there were no easy short-term solutions to the issues at Saint Augustine, but he was determined to move ahead. He decided to prepare a list of options and recommendations to present to Mr. Williams at their regular supervisory meeting next month.

Part **III**

Control

Control through Strategic Management

Carl J. Getto, M.D.

As the twentieth century ends, health care is undergoing a second revolution: not a revolution in theory, but a revolution in the locus of control. One hundred years ago, power was about to shift in a substantial measure away from practitioners and toward medical scientists, but the shift occurred *within* the profession. Doctors won power from doctors. The modern shift cuts more fundamentally into the profession from the outside; it is a wresting of significant amounts of control from the profession by others outside the profession. The modern revolution is a revolution in *accountability*.[1]

The issues of control and accountability are inextricably linked in contemporary health systems. Although it is tempting to focus on a microanalysis of the tactics that might be used to assert control within the environment of an individual hospital or medical practice, it is impossible to view such endeavors apart from the larger system to which they belong. Modern physicians and, in particular, physician executives are accountable for providing high-quality care in a cost-efficient manner to all patients who require it. Moreover, they are responsible for the development and maintenance of a health care system that can merge rapidly changing science and technology into a system of treatment that improves the health of the community. Quality, access, and cost are the primary goals of physicians and physician leaders.

It is important to identify the groups that hold the physician accountable. The physician is accountable first and foremost to the individual patients receiving treatment. Collectively, these patients form the physician's practice, a plan, or a community. Commonly, the community that holds the physician accountable extends beyond the geographical boundaries of the community in which the physician practices.

The physician is also accountable to professional colleagues in a practice group, hospital staff, or professional society. This responsibility extends to all the health professionals with whom the physician practices, and to the institutions in which the physician practices. Although hospitals are the primary institutions that hold the physician accountable, they are but one of the many types of institutions that control the modern practice of medicine. As two of the Part III cases illustrate, insurance companies and their reimbursement plans also affect physicians' behavior.

The issue of control confronts the physician manager with a formidable challenge: to align the goals and the behavior of other professionals with the accountability demanded of them by their constituents. Stephen Shortell has presented compelling evidence for the importance of congruence between hospital goals and physician goals in the success of the hospital. A prime characteristic of successful hospitals and their medical staffs is that they share common goals and operational styles. The successful hospital shares common strategic goals with its medical staff. The two groups can then capitalize on each other's strengths to forge a strategic plan. In this model, control becomes synonymous with accountability. The hospital and the medical staff are accountable to each other for the accomplishment of mutually determined goals through the use of an agreed-upon strategy.[2]

The synergy in such a system results from having all parties participate in the development of the strategic plan. Shortell recommends that to be successful, hospitals must include physicians in strategic planning and decision making. They must share control with their physicians, and the physicians must recognize the importance of cooperating strategically with the hospital. Together the physicians and the hospitals need to monitor their performance and outcomes against the goals and strategy they have selected. When acting congruently, the physicians and hospital will successfully answer to their community.

It is possible to apply this strategy for control to other systems in which the physician executive works. First, a basic agreement on a mutual purpose and the corresponding accountability are established. Second, strategic planning is conducted to define priorities for specific goals and responsibilities. Third, specific techniques for monitoring behavior and performance, such as financial incentives, behavioral reinforcements, and specific negotiations, can be used within the larger context of the collective agreement to cooperate. Often, problems that are attributed to lack of control actually reflect the fact that goals have not been clarified, goals have not been agreed upon by all parties, or conflicting goals have not been adequately prioritized.

The Part III Cases

Controlling magnetic resonance imaging utilization

This case illustrates how multiple constituencies and accountability come into play when a physician executive attempts to exert control. Dr. Sadler's decision is complicated by the following factors:

1. *Allegiance to physician partners.* Dr. Sadler has both a financial responsibility and a responsibility to uphold the quality of medical care that had distinguished this multispecialty group. He was charged with the fiduciary responsibility to see that the group was profitable (in order to pay physician bonuses) and, at the same time, to further the long-term interests of the group in moderating the cost of care.

2. *Allegiance to the traditional "Flexnerian" medical practice.* This dogma determined that science, as interpreted by the individual practitioner, was the predominant force in the practice of medicine. If a physician wanted to practice contemporary, scientific medicine by ordering a magnetic resonance imaging (MRI) scanner, Dr. Sadler had no right to refuse the request.

3. *Accountability to the HMO.* This requires utilization management in order to stay within the bounds of capitation. Also implicit in accountability to an HMO is a responsibility to the community to modulate the cost of medical care.

Case questions

1. Should physicians be held accountable for their own utilization rates of current technology?
2. Comment on the quality assurance issues involved in this case.
3. Compare a capitation rate plan to a fee-for-service plan for the MRI.
4. What issues will cause over- and underutilization of the MRI?
5. What is the effect of advertising the MRI directly to the public?

A new vascular laboratory at St. Giorgio's Hospital

Dr. Jose Graham is faced with the problem that vascular surgery diagnostic imaging has progressed past the technological capabilities at St. Giorgio's. He recognizes the need for new imaging equipment and has three possible ways of bringing it to the hospital. First, he could work within the established corporation. An alternative solution would be to convince the hospital to install the new equipment. A third option would be a joint venture between the hospital and the corporation.

Each of Dr. Graham's alternatives requires that he exert control over individuals and groups by clarifying goals and accountability, including his own. This case illustrates the problems that arise when no one is clearly accountable for the services provided, as when arms-length arrangements are made. In this case, Greenwich Corporation had no responsibility except to run the lab. Its accountability to St. Giorgio's Hospital, the doctors, and the community was limited to operating a vascular lab and breaking even financially. Thus, Dr. Graham faces the need to exert control where there is no accountability.

Case questions

1. Should performance expectations be defined in terms of goal attainment instead of increased budget allocations? If so, how is St. Giorgio's evaluating the vascular laboratory?
2. Some administrators believe that physicians always seem to want "more toys." Is this one of those situations?
3. Is it financially feasible for St. Giorgio's to have a vascular laboratory?
4. What are the control issues present in the case?
5. Suggest an action plan for Dr. Graham.

Physician compensation at Suburban Clinic

Dr. Roberts must control the financial reimbursement system while trying to provide an incentive system under many competing priorities. Among the competing priorities are (1) a productivity incentive for fee-for-service business, (2) a utilization/quality incentive for prepaid services, (3) high-quality care, (4) better community/hospital service, and (5) better clinic development and administration. She has the added tasks of convincing her partners that quality is important in their practice, negotiating an agreement among the partners that quality should factor into their compensation, and defining quality in terms that can be translated into compensation. Dr. Roberts is clearly facing a strategic planning task that goes far beyond a simple compensation scheme.

Case questions

1. What are the benefits of equal income distribution?
2. Why is (or is not) this method of income distribution superior to a production-based model?
3. Should seniority enter into the issue at all?
4. What are the benefits and weaknesses of a staff-model HMO?
5. How can quality enter as a factor of income distribution?

Five departments and a baby

The primary issue for Dr. Johnson is the accountability of Regional Medical Center to the community for providing good care for newborns. It is his responsibility to clarify the priority of newborn care among the goals of the institution. Assuming that the physicians and the hospital administration agree that obstetrical and neonatal care are continued strategic goals, patient care becomes the overriding motivation in forging a solution to the problem. It will be important for Dr. Johnson to determine which parties (among physicians and the administration) have the greatest stake in the goal of maintaining a quality obstetrical/newborn service.

Case questions

1. Who should be in control of neonatal resuscitation?
2. What are the concerns of the hospital?
3. Why is the medical director of the neonatal intensive care unit ineffective?
4. Why is there no accountability for neonatal resuscitation at RMC?

Desert Storm

The Desert Storm case is a good representation of the problems associated with growing economic competition between hospitals and physicians. It also points out some of the problems that can exist with "managing the manager" and in interactions between and amongst the medical staff, the administration, and the hospital board.

"Power" and "control" are two words that immediately come to mind while reading this case, which includes many powerful actors. Mr. Dealer, the new CEO, enters with visions of an expanded hospital role in joint ventures. He has strong views about the subordinate role of physicians in hospital business deals. Yet the physicians from the medical office were involved in several business ventures that were successful. Why should the hospital control all new ventures? The new MRI radiologist knows exactly what he wants. He wants to duplicate the MRI facility that he worked in previously. All actors want things to go the right way . . . *their* way. Is it possible for competing parties to work together in joint ventures?

Case questions

1. Was Mr. Dealer the right man for the job? Comment about the selection process for the CEO position.

2. How should physician loyalty be defined, and by whom? What should the hospital expect from a physician who must choose between the hospital's service and a superior competing service? What should the patient expect?

3. Does competition between hospitals and physicians in some areas preclude collaboration in others? Did the hospital and physician groups do the appropriate stakeholder analysis prior to charting their courses?

4. Who manages the manager? How does the board do its homework to assess the validity of information obtained from administration? How is the administrator performance assessed?

5. Was there a communication problem present in this case? If so, was it amongst physicians, between physicians and the administration, between physicians and the board, between the administration and the board, or between various boards?

6. What was the strategic plan of the administration? How often should an organization review its actions with regard to the mission or the strategic plan, and how flexible should it be in modifying them? How does an organization enlist constructive criticism from respected friends and competitors? Is there a drawback to having leaders surround themselves with those of similar beliefs?

7. How can physicians, management, and board members adapt to a health care environment with shrinking resources and more intense competition?

8. Should the medical staff be structured to address joint venture competition between individual or groups of physicians as they relate to the hospital? In all, none, or selected cases?

9. How should a new administrator with expansionist designs deal with established medical staff members who have already claimed parts of the market?

10. How should management select the individuals or groups to make happy in a win/win/lose situation?

Notes

1. D. M. Berwick, G. A. Blanton, and J. Roessner. *Curing Health Care* (San Francisco: Jossey Bass, 1991), 4.
2. S. Shortell, *Strategic Choices for America's Hospitals* (San Francisco: Jossey Bass, 1990).

Controlling Magnetic Resonance Imaging Utilization

Paul O. Simenstad, M.D., and David A. Kindig, M.D.

Dr. Sadler had a problem, and he needed to decide soon what his solution would be. It was not the most serious issue he had faced in the three years since he became the medical director of Midwest HMO, but the approach he took here would set the tone and course of similar decisions in the future.

Midwest HMO had been quite successful since its inception more than three years ago. It was formed out of a preexisting multispecialty group practice, Midwest Clinic, which had a long history of successful practice in Centerville, a community of about 200,000. Midwest Clinic had grown from six physicians when it began in the 1920s to approximately 140 at the present time.

The clinic had been closely tied to St. Joseph's Hospital, one of the four community hospitals in Centerville, and to the university hospital. As an HMO, the clinic continued to send its patients to St. Josephs when they needed to be hospitalized.

With several major group practices and five hospitals in town, competition had always been present, but the situation changed in 1983 when the state provided strong financial incentives for state and university employees to enroll in capitated plans and mandated capitation for Medicaid recipients. This action stimulated the expansion of the only cooperative HMO in town and the development of HMO plans in the three major clinics and the university hospital. Advertising became intense, particularly during the open enrollment month for state employees. Between 1983 and 1986, the percentage of state employees who were enrolled in HMOs went from 65 percent to 90 percent.

The development of Midwest HMO was a major undertaking for the clinic, but it was made somewhat easier because of the clinic's strong reputation for quality and service and its strong group of physicians. Most patients, except for those with multiple clinic affiliations, would not have to change their physician or location of medical care. However, increased attention had to be paid to controlling costs and utilization, since annual bids would have to be submitted to the state; and state employees were getting accustomed to at least considering their choice of provider based on the monthly rate. The state would pay full capitation rates for individuals who chose the low bid plan, whereas other plans required individuals to add to the state contribution. Table 5.1 shows Midwest HMO's rates compared with rates at other HMOs in the state.

Midwest HMO had done very well in the capitation sweepstakes in Centerville. In the first year, it enrolled 30,000 in the plan; its membership had grown to 58,000 by 1986. Medicaid recipients were initially given the choice of three of the low bid plans; if they did not make a selection within three months, they were assigned by the state to the low bid provider.

Dr. Sadler, an internist, was a past president of the Midwest Clinic and had been active in the administration for many years. He had also been active in the area Blue Shield plan, so he understood insurance and utilization quite well. This knowledge, as well as the respect he enjoyed among his colleagues, made him the logical choice for Medical Director of Midwest HMO, a position that required about half of his work time.

Dr. Sadler's primary job was to control utilization in the capitation practice while maintaining the quality and service that had characterized the clinic in the past. Costs associated with hospitalization accounted for a large proportion of the expenses billed to the HMO. He had achieved control of these charges with a system of inpatient chart reviews, using nurse reviewers who would go over inpatient charts daily and report unusual practices to him the same day. He would act on these reports immediately, sending brief memos or telephoning the HMO physicians to suggest a change in the particular item or to ask for more information about the rationale. He also used this mechanism to provide positive comments on favorable performance. As this system developed, Dr. Sadler was sending out about 125 memos each month.

Dr. Sadler's system had enabled the HMO to reduce its hospital

Table 5.1   1987 Premium Rates by County

	Single			Family		
Plan	State Pays	Employee Pays	Total Premium	State Pays	Employee Pays	Total Premium
Midwest HMO	$73.33	$0.00	$73.33	$190.00	$0.00	$190.00
HMO A	77.02	3.87	80.89	199.35	10.24	209.59
HMO B	71.45	0.00	71.45	182.45	0.00	182.45
HMO C	75.47	0.00	75.47	189.86	0.00	189.86
HMO D	77.02	16.29	93.31	199.35	20.74	220.09

days to about 300 per 1,000 members over the course of the three years. Dr. Sadler felt this figure was about the best that could be achieved given the current case mix. It had been achieved without too much concern on the part of the physicians about control and interference in their practice, but Dr. Sadler knew that this concern was always in the back of their minds. So far, he had been able to increase the incomes of his group each year with moderate bonuses at the end of the year, and he realized that this had a lot to do with the satisfaction of the staff. This year could be different, since the number of new enrollments seemed to have stabilized in the community and at Midwest HMO as well. The competition for inducing existing members to switch clinics was fairly intense, and fees and hospital charges were increasing.

With hospital days at a level that would probably not produce further savings, other items began to attract Dr. Sadler's attention. The explosion in new imaging technology was certainly going to be important in the coming years. The newest technology that was growing in popularity in Centerville was magnetic resonance imaging (MRI). One of the major manufacturers of this equipment was located in the state, so there had been a lot of publicity when MRI was first introduced. The state attempted to regulate the spread of its use by insisting that only two installations could be made in Centerville until the technology was adequately assessed. One MRI unit was initially approved for the university hospital, with most patients being referred there in the early years. State regulations were relaxed somewhat thereafter, which allowed the development of an MRI facility shared by three of the other hospitals in Centerville. This joint venture represented a major departure from the fierce competition that existed between these institutions in almost every other area of activity. It was thought to have occurred as a response to state regulation, the high cost of the equipment, and the competitive threat of the university hospital.

With the additional MRI unit in town and the growing professional acceptance of the technology as a diagnostic aid, the number of procedures performed began to increase. Since Midwest HMO did not have its own MRI, any charges for the procedure had to be paid directly either to the university hospital or to the joint MRI facility. Dr. Sadler had to face the fact that although hospital stays costing the HMO about $800 per day per patient were under control, MRI procedures costing from $500 to $1,000 each were being ordered at an increasing rate. Physicians were pleased with the results and were trying the new technology in many diagnostic situations that had not been fully evaluated. In some instances patients were requesting the procedure even though the physician did not feel it was necessary. At the county medical society meeting, Dr. Sadler learned that the university hospital had begun a system in which each request for MRI was reviewed by a panel of radiologists. He wondered if a similar system would work for the joint facility.

John Jones, the administrator of the joint MRI facility, had approached Dr. Sadler about this. He indicated that he would be willing to negotiate a capitation rate for MRI in order to be sure that all of Midwest's requests for MRI procedures would continue to come to them rather than the university hospital. He said that the data for getting the certificate of need for their facility had indicated that one unit could do about 2,500 procedures per year and therefore could serve a population of about 500,000. He said that he was not sure how MRI would compare with computerized tomography (CT) scannings but that the MRI manufacturers estimated that ultimately 35 percent of CT procedures would be replaced by MRI. No published data existed on ideal or target rates of MRI utilization in large prepaid systems.

In the doctor's lounge at Community Hospital, where most Midwest patients were admitted Dr. Sadler mentioned his conversation with John Jones to one of the neurologists who had been using MRI at an increasing rate. "Sounds good to me, Don," the neurologist replied. "It would allow us to increase utilization of this powerful aid without having to worry about its effect on the HMO. You don't want to have to worry about every single procedure, do you?"

Back in his office at Midwest, Dr. Sadler had three items in his mailbox that were related to this MRI decision. The first was a note from the HMO administrator reminding him that administrative costs were up this year and he needed to submit his list of proposed staffing reductions. The next was a phone message from one of the new internists requesting approval for an abdominal MRI for a patient with recurrent abdominal pain. Finally, there was an article from the local newspaper indicating that two of Midwest's competitors were expected to reduce their bids for state employees this year. Dr. Sadler decided to go home and review all the options available to him so he could make a decision before Monday. Something had to be done, but he didn't see how any more information would help.

A New Vascular Laboratory
at St. Giorgio's Hospital

E. A. Bonfils-Roberts, M.D.

Dr. Jose Graham was appointed Chief of Vascular Surgery at St. Giorgio's Hospital following Dr. Saxon's retirement in 1985. Dr. Saxon had been the head of the section since its creation in 1971.

In his last conversation with Jose Graham, Dr. Saxon talked about his greatest frustration during his tenure in the job—his inability to convince the hospital administration to finance and staff a modern noninvasive vascular laboratory. Since the introduction of this type of laboratory, vascular surgery had expanded into new and innovative areas, and every major institution in the city had established a facility of this type. The equipment necessary to establish a complete laboratory was very expensive and no source of funding other than the administration or the doctors themselves had been found. Dr. Saxon strongly impressed upon Dr. Graham that the issue of the laboratory was going to be of utmost importance if the vascular service was to compete successfully with other institutions. Dr. Graham would need to make every effort to find ways to pay for the equipment.

The hospital is a 1,000-bed tertiary care center owned by the Sisters of New Hope. It is located in a historic area of town, close to the port. Admissions are mainly generated by private practitioners. One-third of the patients are admitted from clinics that serve the poor. The hospital is well known and is considered a leading institution, particularly in the fields of cardiac, vascular, and cancer diseases.

St. Giorgio's was founded by the sisters after they arrived from

Europe in 1830. They also founded one of the oldest nursing schools in the country. Over the years, the hospital established a tradition of excellent patient care. In the past decade, the profound changes brought on by government regulations, Medicare, skyrocketing costs, unions, and increasing salaries had a serious impact on the institution. Moreover, the hospital had engaged over the past few years in an ambitious building and renovation program that resulted in severe financial problems.

Following two episodes of near bankruptcy, the Sisters of New Hope decided to relinquish most of its administrative control to a newly appointed board of trustees. One of the first measures taken by this board was to eliminate the staff managers and bring in a new administration. The attending staff and the new administration clashed from the beginning. It was the perception of the doctors that they were ignored and that their participation in decision making was no longer wanted. The doctors also felt that the managers failed to perceive that hospital income was generated from patients admitted by the physicians in private practice, and not from the indigent population admitted through the clinics.

The attending physicians in private practice voiced their complaints to their respective department heads. The department heads agreed with the issues presented to them, but they decided not to confront the administration. So, the attending staff mounted a strong campaign to have a medical director appointed. They wanted a director who could act as a bridge between the staff and the administration and also control the actions of the chiefs of service. Dr. Alan Knight was appointed as the medical director in 1985.

The History of Vascular Surgery and Noninvasive Techniques

In the early days of vascular surgery, patient assessment was based on careful history and physical examination. Little was available in terms of quantitative evaluation of arterial and venous disease. Angiography was the only means of objective determination of a patient's pathology, and it was not without problems. Cost, discomfort, and the risk of complications associated with the contrast studies precluded angiography from routine use for screening purposes and follow-up evaluations.

The interest in more accurate differential diagnosis, localization of disease, evaluation of severity, and documentation of progression led to the development of noninvasive techniques. By 1980, noninvasive devices with excellent accuracy were developed. For example, imaging is now known to be the best method for visualizing the carotid artery.

In stenosis (narrowing) detection, duplex scanning (imaging) has a superior positive predictive value. In arterial disease of the limbs, segmental arterial pressures and pulse volume recordings provide an objective and quantitative assessment of circulation, and help to confirm the diagnosis made by history and examination. The tests also provide a baseline against which future changes can be measured.

In venous disease, a number of noninvasive studies are available. These studies are so accurate that they have almost replaced venography for the diagnosis of vein insufficiency and occlusion.

St. Giorgio's Vascular Surgery Service and Laboratory

St. Giorgio's vascular surgery service was created in 1971 as an independent unit within the department of surgery. At the time, the use of noninvasive diagnostic methods was in its infancy. By 1983, basic equipment was purchased through funds donated by patients and the vascular surgeons. A professional corporation was created and a full-time technologist was hired. As the years passed, the equipment became obsolete.

By 1985, the vascular surgery service was performing 500 cases per year. All cases were evaluated before and after surgery in the laboratory. In addition, about 600 consultations for noninvasive vascular evaluations were requested annually by other in-hospital services and outside private practitioners. By 1985, when imaging of vessels became popular among vascular surgeons throughout the country, the need to have an imager became essential for the doctors at St. Giorgio's.

The Principals at St. Giorgio's

Jose Graham, M.D., Chief of Vascular Surgery

Dr. Jose Graham was a graduate of South American University. He trained in general surgery at St. Giorgio's and in thoracic and cardiovascular surgery at Olmstead Clinic in the Midwest. After completing his training at Olmstead Clinic, the chief of surgery at St. Giorgio's asked him to return to practice his specialty.

By nature, Dr. Graham was a very independent man and did not agree with many of the ideas held by Dr. Saxon, the chief of vascular surgery at the time he returned to St. Giorgio's. Dr. Graham saw the service as antiquated and conservative, so he concentrated on developing his own practice. He was quite successful and soon began performing most of the vascular surgery cases. When Dr. Saxon retired in 1987,

Dr. Graham was apppointed to replace him, despite Dr. Saxon's open opposition. Dr. Saxon had supported Dr. Seymour Goldstein, his protégé, for the position.

As the chief of vascular surgery, Jose Graham found himself faced with the problem of the vascular laboratory. When the laboratory was founded in 1983, Dr. Graham was not invited to participate in it. Funds came from private donations ($14,000) and contributions from the vascular surgeons ($7,500). This included Dr. Graham's own contribution of $1,500. Very basic equipment was purchased and the laboratory began functioning under the corporate name of Greenwich Vascular Diagnostic Lab, P.C. (Tables 6.1 and 6.2 are financial reports of the laboratory.)

Upon retiring, Dr. Saxon appointed Dr. Seymour Goldstein to become the president of the laboratory. Immediately, Dr. Goldstein began pressing Dr. Graham to persuade the hospital administration to give the lab larger quarters and to consider taking over the laboratory. The issue of acquiring newer, more sophisticated equipment (most importantly, a Duplex imaging device used to study carotid arteries) also came up persistently.

The idea of asking the hospital to take over the ownership and management of the vascular laboratory was an old one. It was clear from the beginning that it would be very expensive to purchase the sophisticated equipment necessary to create a noninvasive study center that could deliver the services required by a large institution like St. Giorgio's and compete for the patients who were going elsewhere. Such a venture would also require highly paid and well-trained technicians.

A hospital takeover was considered the only way to achieve this goal. Over the years, Dr. Graham had advocated this idea. He thought that if the management of the lab and its new equipment were transferred to the department of radiology, he would be able to rid himself of a headache, and the hospital would have a well-run laboratory. He knew that radiology departments in many other institutions were already doing studies of patients with carotid and other peripheral vascular problems. Dr. Graham decided to meet with Dr. Knight, the hospital's newly appointed medical director.

Seymour Goldstein, M.D., President, Greenwich Vascular Diagnostic Lab, P.C.

When Dr. Saxon became the chief of vascular surgery in 1971, he brought in Dr. Seymour Goldstein. Dr. Goldstein was a good surgeon and had a friendly relationship with Dr. Graham. He was well known in the local vascular surgical societies, where he held important political

Table 6.1 Income Statement, Greenwich Vascular Laboratory, P.C.
(1 January 1983 to 31 December 1983)

Income from fees		$14,762.00
Expenses		
Salaries	$12,404.00	
Professional assistants	662.00	
Laboratory and office expenses	3,234.00	
Taxes	831.00	
Legal fees	987.00	
Total expenses		$18,118.00
Net loss		(3,356.00)

Table 6.2 Income Statement, Greenwich Vascular Laboratory, P.C.
(1 January 1988 to 31 December 1988)

Income from fees		$74,400.00
Expenses		
Salaries	$28,004.00	
Laboratory supplies	1,210.00	
Taxes	5,389.00	
Accounting	3,325.00	
Office supplies and expenses	3,052.00	
Billing expenses	9,025.00	
Professional services	4,000.00	
Lease of equipment	20,008.00	
Total expenses		$74,013.00
Net income		387.00

Note: No provision has been made for depreciation of equipment.

positions. He was later appointed as the president of the laboratory by Dr. Saxon, who also declared that Dr. Goldstein should become the chief of vascular surgery upon Dr. Saxon's retirement. Not surprisingly, Dr. Graham's nomination to the position put a strain on the two surgeons' relationship.

Dr. Goldstein agreed that the best course of action regarding the lab was to have the hospital take it over. As a result of his close relationship with Dr. Saxon, he had observed the frustrating process of getting the hospital to consider taking over the management of the lab. He also saw the more serious problem—the medical director's failure to see the need for a vascular laboratory.

By 1986, Dr. Goldstein was ready to consider terminating conversations with the hospital and finding new ways to finance the much needed equipment. He met with a representative of a company that made a Duplex imaging device and other advanced equipment for studying peripheral vascular diseases. Since the company was located only a few miles from the hospital, prompt service was guaranteed, and the representative was willing to arrange financing through a leasing company. A deposit of $12,000 would be sufficient for the company to deliver the machine. At this point, Drs. Graham and Goldstein met with Dr. Knight, who was still considering the possibility of a hospital take-over and the purchase of the machine. Dr. Knight told them that he was going to conduct a feasibility study to decide which machine should be purchased. They informed Dr. Knight of their conversations held with the company representative. They told him that in light of this new option a feasibility study was unnecessary. Their new arrangement would be far superior to those offered by other companies. Nevertheless, Dr. Knight insisted that a study be conducted. Although disappointed, Drs. Graham and Goldstein were encouraged that the administration was finally giving serious consideration to the lab.

Four months later the feasibility study was completed at a great expense, and the investigators recommended the purchase of the same machine that the two doctors had presented to the medical director.

Alan Knight, M.D., Medical Director

Dr. Alan Knight became the medical director at St. Giorgio's in 1985. The position was a new one, and it had become a reality only after long battles between the administration and the directors of services on one side, and the medical staff on the other. The medical staff had wanted somebody who would be able to control the dictatorial powers of the directors and the ineptitudes of the present administration. Once Dr. Knight was appointed, it gradually became clear to the members of the attending medical staff that the cure was worse than the disease.

Dr. Knight's managerial ideas were unfamiliar to the attending physicians. He believed that private practice should no longer exist at St. Giorgio's. He wanted all doctors to be salaried, and he thought about controlling expenses by giving salaries that would be far lower than the income generated by these practitioners. This philosophy coincided with the view of the administration, and it widened the gap between the hospital and its medical staff.

Dr. Knight was not familiar with the role of the vascular laboratory. He failed to understand the significance of noninvasive testing in the management of vascular disease. He wrongly assumed that the noninvasive tests were like those performed by cardiology (e.g., ECG and stress tests) and thought perhaps they had something to do with radiology or some superfluous gimmick of esoteric importance. After he was forced to meet with Drs. Graham and Goldstein on several occasions, he became educated and enlightened on the nature of the tests and their clinical applications. Eventually, he realized that the vascular laboratory would be of great importance to the institution.

Two questions arose in his mind: How could the lab be taken over without incurring any losses? How could the hospital make a profit if the lab was privately run? A quick check with the finance department showed it would be very difficult for the hospital to collect funds from the studies, since these funds would be included in the payments received through the newly established diagnosis-related group (DRG) system.

He decided to contract the services of NFI, Inc. to evaluate equipment needed for the lab (this would further interfere with the two doctors' persistent efforts). He was surprised to learn that the feasibility study suggested that the equipment recommended was the same as originally suggested by the vascular surgeons. It was at this point that Drs. Graham and Goldstein called his office to plan a meeting.

Further Developments

In the meantime, Dr. Goldstein had become frustrated and angry. As the president of the lab, he was reluctant to let the hospital take over its management. He did not want the vascular surgeons to lose control of an important part of the vascular surgery service, especially to the current administration. Noninvasive testing, particularly that of the carotid arteries, required skillful performance by technicians with the active participation of the surgeon ordering the test. If the lab was part of the department of radiology, as Dr. Knight had proposed, Dr. Goldstein feared it would become a small, secondary part of that department—to the detriment of the patients presenting with vascular disease.

Dr. Goldstein felt strongly that the only solution was to purchase the needed equipment through the already existing Greenwich Vascular Diagnostic Lab, P.C. He urged Dr. Graham to become an officer of the corporation. He wanted to finance the project by lease-purchase of the equipment, with himself and Dr. Graham as guarantors. Dr. Graham, in turn, wanted to exercise caution. He still thought there was merit in the idea of radiology taking over operation of the lab. He was also concerned about its financial future. A review of the reports revealed that since its inception, the corporation had barely been able to meet the technician's salary and other expenses. However, he also knew that with new equipment and successful management, revenue would increase tremendously. At least, this was the experience of other area laboratories.

From a political point of view, Dr. Graham did not want to antagonize the medical director. Dr. Knight had told him privately that he should be careful engaging in any venture that was financially dangerous. Dr. Graham made an attempt to get sound advice from the director of surgery but was unable to get the help he needed. He became increasingly disappointed with Dr. Knight. He knew a modern laboratory was an urgent necessity, a fact he could no longer ignore.

Drs. Graham and Goldstein, having grown increasingly frustrated and annoyed, decided that the situation could not continue and called Dr. Knight's office to request a meeting as soon as possible.

Case 7

Physician Compensation at Suburban Clinic

Paul M. Spilseth, M.D.

Dr. Sylvia Roberts is the president of Suburban Clinic, a primary care group practice of 17 doctors, which generates revenue in excess of $4 million a year. Dr. Roberts is an experienced family physician who spends about 75 percent of her time in practice and has administrative duties as the clinic's medical director for the remaining time. She works closely with a lay administrator in running the clinic, and the clinic's governance functions mainly through its operations committee, administrative committee, and HMO committee.

The administrative committee has asked Dr. Roberts for her advice on proposing and implementing a new income distribution formula because Suburban Clinic has been faced with the problem of internal income distribution during the past year. Internal income distribution is an important issue because it influences individual and group behavior.

Dr. Roberts recently completed a class in organizational behavior and is familiar with Abraham Maslow's theories on equity and the hierarchy of needs. She is aware that pay can be a motivator and a demotivator at the same time. She also knows that every group practice must periodically face the potentially destructive decision of how to divide its available net income. Some groups simply split their profits into equal shares, but larger organizations typically enter into more complex arrangements. Factors like variable production, differences in overhead utilization, disproportionate management responsibility, and seniority make it difficult to develop an equation that is satisfactory to all.

Dr. Roberts decides that the first step toward an acceptable method of physician payment is to develop the group's goals, objectives, and mission. With this foundation, the practice can formulate basic criteria for income distribution. The primary goal of physician remuneration must be to achieve equity and fairness for present and future group members. Dr. Roberts sees that all she can hope to achieve is approximate fairness, because there is no method for precisely measuring each member's worth. She also knows that the method of dividing profits must provide proper incentives for the practice's success and growth. Incentives might be provided for increasing gross billings, production, quality of care, or efficiency. However, the formula must be reasonably simple. If the doctors are drawn into an extended debate about many details, the discussion may become more harmful than useful.

Dr. Roberts faces many questions. How should her group design a compensation program to motivate doctors? On what basis should they divide revenues? Should production be a major component? Which should be given more credit—quality or efficiency? Should revenues be divided based on the amount of time spent seeing patients? Should revenues be divided equally? Should intangibles be recognized? Should doctors be paid a salary? Are there other methods that could be used?

History of the Group Practice

In June 1978, the Pine Street Clinic changed its name to Suburban Clinic when it relocated to a new 21,000-square-foot building on the campus of Riverview Hospital in Rivertown. Rivertown is a suburban community located 25 miles from Metro City. The original group moved from a small and crowded building, but the new building was larger than they needed. There were 32 examining rooms, 5 treatment rooms, and 16 private offices for doctors. The facility was functional, of high quality, and residential in character. Many who visited the clinic said it was the nicest clinic they had ever seen.

The building was financed with municipal revenue bonds at a favorable 7 percent interest rate. Shortly after construction of the new building, interest rates skyrocketed and stayed relatively high for the next decade. Soon the group realized the financial difficulties of supporting a new building, especially when it was half full. A recession in 1979 led to decreased patient volumes, increased expenses, and reduced incomes. The business manager left, and the group contracted with a management firm. The group obtained a loan of $150,000 to pay operating expenses, and after several years the difficult situation began to reverse.

The original group consisted of eight physicians (seven family physicians and one surgeon). One family physician left the group in 1980. Between 1979 and 1987, the practice added seven family physicians, three obstetrician-gynecologists, a pediatrician, and an internist. These additions converted the group from a family practice group to a multispecialty group; however, they continued to emphasize primary care.

The new building was only half full, and the clinic realized that the empty space was costly. They felt it would be best to fill the building with their own staff. They considered converting unused space into offices with a separate entrance, but they rejected the idea because the space was new and designed for a single primary care practice. Suburban Clinic elected not to establish multisite practices when its primary site was not fully occupied.

Financial difficulties

Due to financial difficulties in 1979, the group explored alternatives to increase revenues and cut expenses. In November 1979, Metro Clinic, a large group of doctors associated with Metro Hospital, rented about one-third of the space to a specialty care organization called Valley Consultants. This group consisted of urology, dermatology, psychiatry, oncology, gastroenterology, cardiology, pediatrics, and ear, nose, and throat specialists. This arrangement complemented the primary care specialities, but Valley Consultants' volume was not great, and the consultants were not well promoted. Suburban Clinic never fully welcomed Valley Consultants because they saw the consultant group as a competitive threat to their own practice. Eventually, Valley Consultants reduced their space as Suburban Clinic added more of its own physicians. Valley Consultants had provided revenue in the form of rental income at a time of extreme need for Suburban Clinic.

In 1980, Suburban Clinic experienced significant changes with their new accountant, new profit-sharing adviser, and new lay manager. They sold their in-house computer and contracted with a service bureau to handle billing. Another distraction was a lawsuit over a significant portion of the profit-sharing fund that was eventually settled in favor of the clinic.

Beginnings of prepayment

Suburban Clinic's initial experience with prepaid care began in 1978 with an organization called Metropolitan Prepaid Plan (MPP). MPP was an independent practice association of mostly urban doctors from Metro City. The clinic's experience with the plan was brief but unsatisfactory; the group paid money to MPP despite low utilization. This early experience with prepaid care taught the clinic that it could do better independently than grouped with higher-priced, higher-charging urban specialists.

Considering the unused clinic space and the need to grow, the group was receptive to prepaid capitated care. HMOs were an innovative trend that was spreading rapidly in Metro City in the early 1980s. Suburban Clinic was a medium-sized, multispeciality group practice. There were large employers in the area, and state and federal laws were changing to make prepaid care viable. So, in 1981, Suburban Clinic began its first risk experience with prepaid care with Statewide HMO and Universal Health Care. Initial contracts covered only ambulatory care and not hospital care.

First experiences with prepaid care caused some anxiety among physicians. One of the first HMO patients had an unusual mesothelioma that required expensive radiation therapy and hospitalization, which resulted in high costs to the group. Group leaders worried about adverse selection and high utilization. But the early experiences with prepaid care were financially sound, which surprised the skeptical physicians. HMO membership grew rapidly.

General Windows was the area's largest employer, and in 1982 Universal Health Care offered General Windows an HMO contract that included a reduced premium if Suburban Clinic was the exclusive provider. The plan was attractive to employees and management. The contract brought significant numbers of new patients to the clinic, and many patients transferred from the competing primary care group. The doctors and staff became increasingly comfortable with prepaid care. They understood that they could provide needed services in an efficient manner without incurring losses. Hospital usage decreased, but the doctors and staff perceived an increase in patient demand for clinic visits. The clinic members realized that they could not treat mental health and chemical dependency, so in 1984 they began to contract these services out on a capitated arrangement to a mental health group.

In 1983 the group began to take full risk in their HMO contracts for all medical care, including hospitalization, emergency room, and referral services. The clinic was responsible for all medical care expenses for outpatient, inpatient, referrals, ambulance, and mental health and chemical dependence services. Payments were $27 per member per month. Even with this comparatively low payment, the clinic showed a 7.9 percent surplus when compared with fee-for-service plans. The clinic began to search for more prepaid business. They realized they were ideally positioned to grow and prosper in this changing environment.

In 1984 they began a relationship with Good Health Plan (GHP). GHP is a large, staff-model HMO that started in the 1930s. They chose the Suburban Clinic as one of two groups in their initial HMO network. The clinic again experienced significant growth in membership in a relatively short period of time. In 1985 a Medicare HMO was offered through Good Health, the first HMO offered to individuals rather than groups. The first two years of the Medicare experience were a financial disaster, but this reversed after the long-ignored needs of the elderly were met.

By January of 1988 the prepaid membership in the three HMOs was 7,624 patients. Prepaid revenues represented half of the gross revenues.

Income distribution

The mechanism for physician payment at Suburban Clinic evolved over a ten-year period. Revenues from all sources were first allocated to pay operating expenses such as overhead, administrative costs, and ancillary services. The remainder was divided according to a formula. Initially, 50 percent of the net was divided equally, and 50 percent was divided based on production. As obstetrics specialists were added, increases were made in the production portion to accommodate them. From 1980 through 1986, the income distribution system was 60 percent based on production, 30 percent divided equally, and 10 percent by seniority. The seniority portion was divided equally after five years in the practice. For the first five years, 2 percent of the seniority portion was added to physician reimbursement each year. After the fifth year, the full 10 percent of the seniority portion was added. In 1987 the formula was changed to 70 percent production, 20 percent equal, and 10 percent seniority.

Production was measured by gross billings, bookings, and services. Production credit for ancillary services (laboratory and x-ray) was traditionally included in gross billings. The group dropped lab and x-ray credit in 1988 in an attempt to decrease the incentive to use laboratory resources for prepaid patients.

Negotiations for a New Distribution System

Dr. Roberts has discussed income distribution issues with several doctors. She has studied the numbers, and she has compared notes with other medical directors. In 1986 the total gross production for the 13 senior physicians was $2,782,492. After paying expenses, the amount available for distribution to physicians was $1,112,996. Now Dr. Roberts must take into account the physicians' perspectives on the issue. She asks the physicians to review and discuss the distribution figures for 1986 (see Table 7.1). Her ensuing conversation with the doctors results in a lively debate.

The income distribution for the group is complicated by earnings obtained outside of clinic time, such as occupational medicine, medical directorships of nursing homes, and working in the emergency room. Dr. Smith had proportionately higher income compared to production because he has outside income from a community industry.

Dr. Miner, the highest-producing specialist, has been doing some figuring and feels he is getting less than his share. Dr. Miner produced $281,721 in billed charges and Dr. Jones produced $156,466. Dr. Miner has added these two gross production numbers and subtracted approximately 60 percent for expenses, including rent, professional liability, salaries, and costs of purchased services for HMO patients. The remaining 40 percent was wages and benefits to physicians ($175,275 in this example). He calculated that the 30 percent equal portion, including seniority, was $52,582, and the 70 percent production portion was $122,693. Table 7.2 shows his income distribution figures for the two physicians.

Dr. Miner points out to Dr. Jones that even though the 1986 formula was weighted in favor of production, Dr. Jones's income in relation to billed charges was higher than his ratio. In other words, Dr. Miner received 37 percent of billed charges as income, whereas Dr. Jones received 45 percent of gross billings.

Dr. Jones responds by showing that Dr. Miner's figures are in error. In 1986, the formula stated that the equal share/seniority amount was 40 percent. After subtracting 60 percent for expenses, the remaining 40 percent was for physician salary and benefits (profit sharing, insurance, and other benefits), and benefits totaled 20 percent of total compensation. In this case, $35,055 is the equal split amount per physician, and not the $26,291 used by Dr. Miner. Dr. Jones determines that his salary should have been $72,609 and Dr. Miner's $102,666.

Dr. Jones believes that the formula was fair because each doctor in a cohesive group works equally to provide efficient care. When a doctor is working, regardless of what he or she was doing, that work contributes equally to the welfare of the organization. Dr. Jones points out that his training as a pediatrician was just as difficult as Dr. Miner's obstetrics training. The phone calls he handles require as much judgment as doing high-priced procedures, yet the phone calls produce no income.

Drs. Anderson and Johnson argue that they provide referrals and

Table 7.1   1986 Income Distribution

Doctor	W-2	Wages and Benefits	Gross Production
Smith	$77,005	$ 75,392	$171,443
Jones	57,438	71,798	156,466
Olson	60,351	75,438	171,634
Roberts	62,310	77,887	181,838
Anderson	60,211	75,264	170,908
Johnson	67,835	84,794	210,616
White	71,322	89,152	228,775
Harris	72,824	91,030	236,601
Green	75,782	94,727	252,006
Wright	73,991	92,489	242,680
Keller	77,327	96,658	260,051
Bush	69,205	86,507	217,753
Miner	81,487	101,859	281,721

Table 7.2   Distribution of 1986 income for Dr. Miner and Dr. Jones (Dr. Miner's calculations)

	Dr. Miner	Dr. Jones
Billed charges	$281,721	$156,466
Equal shares portion	26,291	26,291
Productivity portion	78,881	43,810
Total income	$105,172	$ 70,101
Percent of income to billed charges	37%	45%

take calls for the surgical specialties. As part of the group practice, they think they should share in a portion of the overall profits generated from higher-priced procedures.

Dr. White notes that one solution to the dilemma of distribution of funds in a mixed fee-for-service/prepaid (FFS/PPD) group is simply to pay each member of the group on a prearranged salary. This employee-type relationship would be attractive to those new in practice and to those desiring part-time practice. A salary distribution system in a prepaid group would be in the best interest of the patient. The doctor-patient relationship would be strengthened. There would be no incentive for the physician to overutilize or underutilize services. Such an arrangement would remove the potential for conflict of interest, and overcharging would not be rewarded. When a new and difficult procedure became less difficult and commonly performed, charges for the procedure should decrease appropriately. Participation in hospital and community activities would be recognized financially because incentives to increase billings would be removed.

Dr. Miner argues that if production incentives were removed, the potential for inefficiency would be greater. A salaried physician is rewarded financially for time spent working, but not for efficient use of time. Salaried physicians might overuse ancillaries to minimize their own work, or refuse to see patients because it is more personally satisfying to care for a small number of patients than to supervise the care of more patients. In addition, the amount of revenue distributed to physicians is not predictable from year to year, so establishing a salary amount would be impossible. The clinic liquidates almost all of its funds at year end to avoid corporate taxes.

Dr. White suggests that if production were rewarded on the prepaid side, there would be potential for physicians to encourage patients to return for marginally discretionary needs or to do procedures with questionable merit. The patient would bear no out-of-pocket expense, and the physician would be rewarded on a production basis. This production system evolved from the fee-for-service environment, but now it works against efficiency on the prepaid side.

What Should Dr. Roberts Do?

Dr. Roberts thinks the group must maintain some production portion in the formula, but she feels she should devise a system to recognize quality and efficiency as well. The clinic has just started a quality assurance committee, but so far the physicians have little interest. If she could tie quality of patient care to physician pay, she feels she could generate more enthusiasm for increasing quality. Insurers, HMOs, and corporations select their contracts based on quality of services. The clinic should understand how to improve quality of care and should use it as a selling point.

The problem of internal distribution of revenue is complicated by the pluralistic environment of differing payment sources. In addition, there should be some way to recognize intangible contributions to the practice, such as participation in group and hospital committees, community activities, medical society responsibilities, and writing/teaching at the nearby university.

You have been a friend of Dr. Roberts since medical school. You have just completed a master's degree in administrative medicine at State University. Dr. Roberts asks for your advice and direction regarding income distribution in her group.

Case 8

Five Departments and a Baby

Kenneth C. Cummings, M.D.

Robert Johnson, M.D., the new director of medical affairs at Regional Medical Center (RMC), who had recently been recruited from a similar position in another institution, received an urgent telephone call from an agitated staff obstetrician.

DR. SIMONS: I just thought I'd let you know that we may have a major problem on our hands. Within the next hour or so, I'll be taking a complicated patient of mine to the delivery room and there is a signifi-cant probability that the newborn will need resuscitation. I've just been told that neither a pediatrician nor an anesthesiologist will be available. There are lots of professionals around here that should be able to help. I'm not concerned about liability or reimbursement or staffing. I want you to do something about this NOW!

DR. JOHNSON: Thanks for letting me know about this. I can certainly understand your concern. I will check into the matter and get back to you shortly.

Dr. Johnson contacted Dr. Gina Miro, chair of the Department of Anesthesiology, and summarized the problem for her.

DR. MIRO: This is no surprise to me. We have struggled with this prob-lem for ten years and I have just about had it! For the patient's benefit, I will rearrange our coverage of the operating room and make an anes-thesiologist available, but our patience is running thin. You need to understand that we don't see this as our problem.

The alteration in the OR schedule was needed to provide anesthesia coverage for the obstetrician, who, as circumstances evolved, did call for the assistance of an anesthesiologist. The new mother and infant did well, but it was obvious to Dr. Johnson that this problem concerning the availability of resuscitators for emergency resuscitations at birth could not be allowed to continue.

Background

Regional Medical Center is a 300-bed, acute care community hospital located in the rapidly growing southern section of a large midwestern city. Founded in 1874, it is one of the oldest private hospitals west of the Mississippi. The hospital relocated from the inner city to its present location in 1977, and it enjoys an excellent reputation in the community for the quality of care it provides and the quality of its medical staff and nursing. RMC also has a reputation for innovation in the community. It introduced a helicopter service for trauma patients in 1978; it offered the first aging services program in the state; it developed the first three-dimensional color reconstructed computerized tomographic capability in the Midwest; and it was the first hospital in the area to obtain a mobile magnetic resonance imager.

The nearest competitor to RMC is an aggressive for-profit hospital that shares many of RMC's medical staff. This competitor has recently made plans to develop a Level III neonatal intensive care unit (NICU) and to hire and relocate several neonatologists.

The area is blessed with a large children's hospital, which is located 30 minutes from RMC. The chief of neonatology at the children's hospital is also on staff at RMC and is held in high regard.

The labor and delivery area at RMC is modern, well equipped, and well staffed, and the adjoining nursery has a Level II NICU that is also well equipped and well staffed. Approximately 150 patients deliver each month, and some form of neonatal resuscitation is needed on a daily basis. Regarding neonatal resuscitation, no significant untoward events have occurred.

Since the hospital was relocated, an unpaid, board-certified neonatologist, whose office is located in the adjoining medical office building, has served as the medical director of the NICU. He very much enjoys general pediatrics as well as neonatology, he is well liked, and he participates on a hospital board committee. Recently, he has become annoyed by frequent calls for help from the delivery room when no one else is available.

Stakeholders

The patient

The patient is the hospital's primary stakeholder. Over the past several decades, seemingly miraculous technological and therapeutic advances have been made in the pediatric subspecialty of neonatology. Concurrent with these new and efficacious treatment modalities there has evolved an inflexible societal attitude that when there is a suboptimal patient outcome, someone (doctor, nurse, or hospital) must have erred. Because awards for damages in pediatric malpractice suits are based upon a lifetime of continuing medical and custodial needs, plus the presumed loss of a lifetime of earnings, the economic awards in successfully prosecuted suits are staggering for physicians, hospitals (under a legal theory of corporate negligence), and their insurers.

The obstetrician

The obstetricians at RMC are board certified and enjoy an excellent professional reputation. Although they are busy, they have experienced a loss of patients to family practitioners who also provide obstetric services. There is considerable tension between the obstetrics-gynecology and family practice departments in the areas of competition, reimbursement, and credentialling. Family practitioners compete aggressively with obstetricians but also need them to consult in complicated cases. The business overhead in each of the specialties has risen more rapidly than the national inflation rate, and obstetric malpractice insurance premiums approach $100,000 annually.

The obstetrician knows that, in the delivery room, he or she is responsible for everything that occurs during the delivery process. Not uncommonly, the mother needs personal medical attention just at the time the newborn infant requires intensive resuscitative therapy. A major problem for an obstetrician or pediatrician is that, although intensive neonatal resuscitation may be anticipated following a complicated pregnancy, it is also commonly required following an otherwise uncomplicated delivery. For this reason, the obstetrician insists that another professional be immediately available.

The family practitioner

As noted above, some family practitioners want to deliver their own pregnant patients' babies. If they possess the required specialty board certification along with training in obstetrics, they are allowed to deliver in uncomplicated cases. Of course, their malpractice insurance is much increased if they practice obstetrics. Their circumstances are slightly different than those of the obstetrician because family practitioners also expect to become the physician for the newborn infant. Tension exists between the family practitioner and pediatrician because both compete for the same pediatric patients. The pediatrician desires referrals of very sick children from the family practitioner and the family practitioner needs the ready availability of consultative backup from the pediatrician. If both the mother and the newborn need professional attention, the family practitioner again must have professional backup immediately available.

The pediatrician

For many reasons, some pediatricians choose to perform neonatal resuscitation while others do not. Beyond personal interest, a number of factors may weigh into this decision: increased malpractice liability for pediatricians who do neonatal resuscitation, loss of newborn patients for their practice if they do not, and a major negative impact on their office schedule if they are called to the delivery room to wait for a possible resuscitative need. Because the pediatrician's practice is almost entirely office based, the impact of increased waiting room time for patients is critical. Although the pediatrician is a professional and the patient comes first, it is also true that third party insurers tend to reimburse poorly (currently averaging approximately $100) for resuscitation, which is a negative factor in the pediatrician's (and family practitioner's) consideration of whether or not to offer the service.

In addition, pediatricians must maintain good working relationships with obstetricians, who frequently are sources of new patients for their practice. If the obstetrician has an urgent need and the pediatrician does not fulfill it, the obstetrician is likely to look to another pediatrician, not only for the immediate need but also regarding future referrals.

In the RMC area, the medical community appears adequately staffed with neonatologists, so a new neonatologist would have to take market share from those already established. This too is a deterrent to pediatricians considering neonatal resuscitation services.

The anesthesiologist

Anesthesiologists or certified registered nurse anesthetists (CRNAs) are commonly called upon because they are experts in resuscitation and because, due to their other duties, they are almost always in the hospital. They face liability, reimbursement, and scheduling issues that are similar to those of the other physicians. Recently, the American Society of Anesthesiologists has determined that neonatal resuscitation is not part of the anesthesiologists's primary hospital role. Not surprisingly, anesthesiologists are even less interested in providing neonatal resuscitative services because they see this change in role definition as increasing their potential liability. In addition, they are angered at being left "holding the bag" when a newborn needs resuscitation and no one else is available. Nevertheless, the anesthesiologists at RMC have never refused to provide the service.

The department of nursing

Nurses are routinely trained to provide only initial, noninvasive neonatal resuscitation. It is conceivable that, in an emergency situation in which only the nurse and the obstetrician are in the delivery room, the nurse might be called upon to provide resuscitative assistance for the newborn until help arrives. During this interim period, the infant might be at increased risk, and delivery room personnel would most certainly be greatly stressed. Nurses might be called upon to provide services that are not in their position descriptions, for which they are not trained, not certified, and not directly supervised. Although covered legally as employees of the hospital, nurses in this situation do experience an increase in malpractice liability exposure. The nurses at RMC are ambivalent about providing this service (even after training), but they see it as an opportunity for better patient care and for a more significant role in the delivery process.

RMC does have an attractive career advancement program for nurses, which provides reward for additional training. Further, the department of nursing is aggressively pursuing the concept of shared governance for nurses, whereby staff nurses would be allowed more autonomy and personal decision-making authority.

The hospital administration

The hospital administration must balance complex and often conflicting goals of the various stakeholders when solving complex problems such as this. The administration represents the board of directors, which is ultimately responsible for everything that happens in the hospital. The hospital must first protect its patients. Because of the legal concept of corporate negligence, hospitals are frequently named in malpractice suits even though the medical care provided by the physician is principally at issue. The hospital offers an additional "deep pocket" and, because of the legal concept of joint and several liability that is commonly operative in the United States, it may eventually pay the majority of the damages awarded in a successfully prosecuted malpractice suit.

The appropriate management of nurses and their work environment is critical to the mission of RMC (e.g., nurse retention) as well as to maintain positive working relationships with staff physicians. Thus far, RMC has been very successful in recruiting and retaining nurses. However, local competitors have recently initiated a nurse recruiting effort, offering both monetary and nonmonetary inducements.

The medical director of the NICU

As stated above, the medical director of the NICU is a board-certified neonatologist who also has an active practice in general pediatrics and is one of two neonatologists on staff (the other being the chief of neonatology at the local children's hospital). He has given general direction to the NICU for approximately ten years without pay and has recently been stressed by an increasing number of emergency calls to the delivery room when no other resuscitator was available. Further, he has recently expressed the desire for fundamental, although not well-defined, changes in his relationship with the NICU.

This physician very much enjoys the practice of general pediatrics and has a large practice of significant importance to the hospital. Further, he is a senior member of the medical staff and recently declined a request to become president-elect of the medical staff. He also participates on a hospital board committee. He has two nonneonatologist pediatrician partners, is otherwise happy with his practice, and is not interested in taking on another associate.

Previous Solution

Approximately one year ago, a list was developed of pediatricians and family practitioners interested in performing neonatal resuscitation. Any pediatrician or family practitioner not on the list was required to select someone on the list so that, if the nonresuscitating physician's patient delivered and neonatal resuscitation was required, the previously identified resuscitator would be called. In addition, initial certification and biannual recertification in neonatal advanced life support (NALS) were required of all resuscitators, along with board certification in their clinical specialty.

Although every effort was made by the resuscitators to respond quickly when called, the problem persisted because many of the resuscitators' offices were a 10- to 30-minute drive from the hospital. The delay frequently resulted in the need to call an anesthesiologist or the medical director of the NICU. The NICU and delivery room nurses were becoming increasingly anxious about the difficulty in getting timely resuscitative backup. It caused an awkward professional circumstance and created concern for the welfare of the newborn infants.

The issue was finally brought to a critical point when the head of the anesthesiology department, out of frustration and to precipitate a solution, announced that her department, in the near future, would no longer provide neonatal resuscitative backup.

Desert Storm

Alan R. Altman, M.D.

White Dunes Hospital is a 350-bed, not-for-profit community hospital located in the Southwest, which developed a for-profit arm to compete with neighboring Sands Hospital. In 1987, the hospital opened a cardiac surgery program. Two years later, it was still floundering. Attempts made to coerce the medical staff to use this program had led to strife and divisiveness. The medical staff was divided into two factions with the private doctors in independent practice on one side and the few contract physicians who enjoyed a longtime affiliation with the hospital on the other.

At least 20 of the private practitioners had gone into private practice when the multispecialty clinic they belonged to was forced into bankruptcy. Many of the subspecialists practiced both at White Dunes Hospital and at Sands Hospital. Sands, a 230-bed facility located approximately ten miles from White Dunes Hospital, had boasted an excellent cardiac surgery program for more than 13 years. Most patients preferred to receive medical care in their own community rather than travel even ten miles, except when they need certain specialized services such as heart surgery and orthopedics.

The Joint Venture History

In 1985, White Dunes Hospital performed a feasibility study that showed physician interest in a medical office building joint venture on the hospital campus. A group of 32 physicians had expressed interest and had appointed five people to negotiate with the hospital and develop the project. After several months, a negotiated agreement was reached, but at the last minute the hospital administrator and chair of the board could not decide whether the hospital was "getting anything" by entering the venture. This led to physician distrust of both the administration and the board. Subsequently, a two-acre parcel of land across the street from the hospital was purchased by the physicians, and in 1989 a medical office building was constructed to house 22 busy private practitioners.

A separate partnership, Ancillary Services, was also formed and included a full-service clinical laboratory. Referrals were sent outside to labs and to the hospital when possible. The hospital received approximately $10,000 worth of work from the laboratory every month. Outpatient laboratory studies previously had been done by other independent laboratories, and the hospital had no significant outpatient market.

Ancillary Services also included a radiology suite in which state-of-the-art equipment was used. The clinical laboratory and radiology suites were located in the new medical office building complex. A cardiology service, also part of the partnership, was located in the building and was directed by a Harvard-trained, board-certified cardiologist. Each member of the building as well as each member of the Ancillary Services partnership remained independent, and no efforts were made to influence referrals between physicians or to various facilities. Great care was taken to conform the Ancillary Services partnership to all existing state and federal laws. Profits from Ancillary Services were divided strictly based upon investment, and not by referral. The Ancillary Services radiology section consisted of three of the ten White Dunes Hospital radiologists who rotated to the outpatient service on a weekly basis. These individuals were selected by the Ancillary Service partners because of their proven superior abilities as well as excellent relationships with staff and patients. The decision to use hospital radiologists rather than recruit an independent radiologist was made after much deliberation. In part it was a political concession to try to preserve good relationships between the hospital, hospital contract physicians, and physicians in the building. Prices charged for services were 10 percent lower on the average than the hospital outpatient charges, except for fixed Medicare charges.

The Ancillary Services partnership had originally planned to include a computerized tomography (CT) unit as part of the radiology unit. In an effort to preserve and enhance relationships with the hospital, as well as to avoid duplication of capital expense, negotiations were held with the hospital regarding a joint venture for use of an existing hospital outpatient CT scanner. An agreement was reached whereby the partnership bought into the existing CT scan unit at 50 percent of its present value, and a new partnership was constructed that consisted of 50 percent ownership by the hospital and 50 percent ownership by the Ancillary Services group. This was a one-year partnership with the option to terminate or to continue or enhance the partnership after a year.

The New Administrator

Mr. Sage Dealer was hired as the new chief executive officer at White Dunes Hospital early in 1989. He had moved from a similar position at a slightly larger hospital where he had confided to one colleague that he was "just burnt out by the physicians." He had been selected over three other candidates, primarily because of his reputation as a doer, as someone who could create joint projects and help bond physicians and hospitals. The search committee, which included board members and some medical staff, were impressed by his energy, charisma, and assertiveness. He had been a hospital administrator for 15 years, serving for five years at each of his last two jobs.

In his initial period at White Dunes Hospital, Mr. Dealer scheduled appointments with virtually every doctor on the staff and had long and frank discussions with them regarding the hospital, its functioning, and the various political factions. He expressed in no uncertain terms that he would advocate whatever was in the hospital's best interest.

Frequent informational meetings were held by the administration and staff with nursing and medical staff, and there were informal wine and cheese gatherings as well. Mr. Dealer was successful in gaining the confidence of several physicians, whom he then gave more influence by having them appointed to various strategic committees and in some cases to positions on the board. The chief of staff, an anesthesiologist, was offered a contract for anesthesiology services, which previously had been offered only on a fee-for-service, independent basis. The chief of staff became a close ally of the administration.

Over the ensuing months there was a general feeling that the hospital itself was looking better. There were also plans for expansion, growth, and an enhanced image in the community. Mr. Dealer joined the hospital in time to negotiate and finalize the CT agreement. At the same time, an agreement was reached to make the hospital's for-profit arm a passive general partner in the entire Ancillary Services project as well as a purchaser of one limited partner share. Mr. Dealer had said that his intent in completing the joint venture was to show that the hospital could in fact develop a successful joint venture with physicians. His grand plan was to try to develop a larger joint venture involving all or most of the physicians on the medical staff, and to merge the existing CT partnership into a larger one. It was agreed that the hospital management would continue to administer the outpatient CT operation, and the physician management would administer the outpatient Ancillary Services partnership. There would be meetings and communication between the two at regular intervals. Concerns were raised by the physician group regarding the potential shunting of outpatient CT work to the hospital inpatient unit or to a freestanding mobile unit on hospital grounds, so the hospital would benefit 100 percent from those scans rather than share the profits on a 50 percent basis with physicians. Provisions were added to the agreement to address these problems.

The ancillary services project was quite successful. The joint CT venture also was extremely successful, despite the hospital's poor management of the project. Frequently, when office staff called to schedule a CT scan, they were told there was a one-week wait, despite the fact that only 4 to 6 scans were being done each day on a machine that could easily handle 12 to 14 scans per day. In direct meetings and written correspondence, the physicians involved in management of the ancillary services project pointed out that the unit was not performing at maximum efficiency.

The Administrator in Action

When Mr. Dealer took the job at White Dunes Hospital, he was able to gather information regarding the structure and political climate at the hospital. He realized that the previous administration had a favored relationship with a very small number of contract physicians. These physicians had been given very favorable long-term contracts, which were renewed on an interim basis without serious risk of displacement by new competition.

The physicians favored by the cardiology, radiology, and pathology contracts had been community residents for many years and were instrumental in the growth of the hospital by obtaining contributions from prominent citizens.

There seemed to be two groups of physicians. One group was heavily influenced by the hospital cardiology contract physicians, the other by the busy independent physicians in private practice, many of whom were in the new medical office building. The leadership of the latter group was divided between three physicians: a primary care physician, a medical subspecialist, and a surgeon. The three had been leaders in the development of the medical office building project, and the surgeon had been a pioneer in developing an outpatient surgery center immediately adjacent to the medical office building.

Mr. Dealer felt that private practice was most likely going to be replaced by a managed care system, and his hope was to develop such a system at the hospital to compete successfully in the new medical environment. He thought that physicians would fare better under this arrangement. To this end, he devoted time and resources to the further advancement of a fledgling hospital-related independent practice association (IPA), and the hospital employees were "coerced" economically into changing their medical insurance to become the first large group under this IPA. Many of the primary care physicians in the medical office building did not join this association, which led to an ongoing rift between the administration and the physicians across the street.

The primary care physicians, as well as some of the subspecialists, felt that their office building and the ancillary services project were appropriate responses to changing times and changing environments. Complete physician control was certainly preferable to having a hospital-controlled operation. The hospital, with its many boards and committees, had developed a reputation over many years as an inflexible organization, one that was unable to accomplish necessary change.

The hospital services, while adequate, were never thought to be totally efficient, amiable to physicians and patients, or innovative in any way. Most of the independent physicians had very busy, active practices and did not need or want an additional patient load at discounted rates. Theirs was a relatively large physician-run IPA that allowed people their choice of hospital based upon the physician they chose, whereas the hospital IPA restricted hospitalization to White Dunes Hospital.

Mr. Dealer was unsuccessful in recruiting the most popular primary care physicians into the IPA, although a number of the surgical and subspecialty staff did join. After attempts to entice these physicians to join the hospital IPA, Mr. Dealer decided to change his strategy. He realized that the previous medical clinic, which had folded, was not well thought of by many of the current physicians. Mr. Dealer began referring to the physicians in the medical office building as a group, and he equated them with the previous medical clinic when he spoke with other independent physicians on staff. He also referred to these physicians as disloyal because they were hurting the hospital by having competing ancillary services. He tried to erode the partnership by wooing away some individual members. He wanted to develop an outpatient cancer center, and he contracted with an outside group to begin development, undaunted by the fact that there was a great deal of opposition from both the oncologists and the general medical staff.

The physicians became polarized into a smaller group of favored physicians (those working with the administration), a group of unfavored physicians (physicians in the medical office building), and a larger group of physicians who were being recruited by the administration to join forces with the hospital in a new expansion effort.

Mr. Dealer recognized that in the long run he would need new physicians, both in primary care and in certain subspecialties. The hospital began a recruitment process and, without significant staff input, started bringing in primary care physicians without serious screening and without choosing candidates with special expertise. The hospital helped them get settled in the community by providing office space and certain guarantees. An oncologist was brought in to head the cancer center. A much needed infectious disease person was recruited. Some of these actions were severely upsetting to the medical staff as it appeared obvious that the hospital was recruiting physicians who were only needed to divert market share away from existing physicians and to be loyal to the hospital in terms of sending ancillary service work to the hospital services.

Problems persisted in the fledgling heart surgery program. The heart surgeon, although a good one, had problems relating to various physicians and was quite careful in his patient selection. He had a tendency to blame any adverse occurrence on the medical or nursing staff and not on himself. He was often abrupt and was apt to change his opinion and stories frequently. He felt that the medical staff was obligated to refer their patients to him. He shared this opinion with the administration, and pressures were exerted on physicians who were sending their patients elsewhere for cardiac surgery to change their referral pattern and use the White Dunes hospital heart surgeon. However, it was generally recognized that the heart surgery program at Sands Hospital was superior. Physicians were forced to decide whether to send their patients to the better program and be "disloyal" to the hospital, or to utilize White Dunes Hospital and be less loyal to their patients. The hospital board was influenced by administration and supported efforts to compel physicians to use the hospital service. Attempts were made to tie emergency room call privileges for cardiologists to a mandatory use of the hospital heart surgeon. Mr. Dealer unilaterally removed the emergency room privileges of one cardiologist who continued to use the competitive heart surgeon, even though the cardiologist also occasionally used the hospital heart surgeon. The hospital was sued by this physician and the courts decided in favor of the physician. Nevertheless, the hospital administrator and the board did not change and continued to push their policy.

The Nursing Service and the Union

Although the previous board had taken some steps to reverse the poor financial status of the hospital, the new administrator continued to make significant cuts in staffing. The nursing staff was very unhappy with administration. They felt that the administration was dishonest and unappreciative of patient care issues. This led to discussions about the formation of a union. A vote was held and the union was defeated by four votes, which the administration viewed as a great victory. Low morale led to an exodus of experienced nurses to other institutions.

The MRI Joint Venture

The hospital had one MRI unit and rotated the hospital radiologists through it. Many of the radiologists had no significant background or training with MRI, and many of the interpretations were inadequate. There was often a two-week wait. Many physicians did not use the MRI because of the combination of lack of accessibility and lack of competence in interpreted results. A total of 10 to 12 scans were being done daily. Since the hospital was a regional trauma center, many of the scans were on inpatients. During this period of time, a radiologist with expertise in MRI and CT, who had successfully operated an MRI outpatient unit that competed with several hospital outpatient units, expressed a strong interest in relocating to the White Dunes Hospital area. He knew there was a significant community need for MRI expertise, which influenced his decision to relocate. He initially had discussions with physicians in the medical office building to see if there would be room in their facility for him to open up an MRI unit. The physician leadership decided this would be an opportunity to build bridges. A joint venture was developed by the physicians and the radiologist to incorporate a new outpatient MRI unit with the hospital MRI facility. The preliminary details are outlined in Tables 9.1 and 9.2.

Mr. Dealer was furious when he first heard about the project. He was at a meeting in an adjacent community and overheard a friend having a conversation about an MRI joint venture being developed in the White Dunes area. When he returned to his office he had his secretary place a call immediately to Dr. Dalton, the doctor who he'd heard had been responsible for the collaboration. Despite the fact that it was the middle of office hours, Mr. Dealer insisted that the doctor be interrupted to speak with him.

"Dalton, I thought we were partners. How dare you put together

Table 9.1   Resource and Use Requirements for Proposed Outpatient
MRI Unit

Project Requirements	Total Project	Cash Up Front
New Equipment (freestanding)		
MRI unit purchase	$1,500,000	$ 300,000
Used Equipment (hospital based)		
GE MRI unit (1.6T) purchase	1,800,000	360,000
Sales tax (6%)	$ 198,000	$ 39,600
Total (major equipment)	$3,498,000	$ 699,600
Other Expenses		
Equipment upgrades	100,000	100,000
Buildout for new equipment	500,000	250,000
Minor medical equipment	50,000	50,000
Office equipment	20,000	20,000
Furnishing	20,000	20,000
Telephone system	10,000	10,000
Computer	25,000	25,000
Inventory	15,000	15,000
Signage	10,000	10,000
Outside legal services	10,000	10,000
Working capital	155,550	155,550
Organization and development	60,000	60,000
Brokerage fees	90,000	90,000
Total (other expenses)	$1,065,550	$ 815,550
Complete project	$4,563,550	$1,515,150
Complete project cost		$4,563,550
Cash required		1,515,150
Balance to be financed		$3,048,400
	Amount of Contribution	Total Contributions
General partners (2)	$7,575	$ 15,150
Limited partners (300)	$5,000	$1,500,000

a joint MRI venture without even letting me know about it. I had to hear about this in another community! I am disappointed in your behavior. You know my position. The hospital must be the one formulating the joint ventures. Your group of physicians will certainly be welcome

Table 9.2 Projected Volume and Revenue for Proposed Outpatient MRI Unit (based on 260 workdays per year)

Category	Current	Year 1	Year 2	Year 3	Year 4	Average (Years 5–10)
Volume per Day						
MRI (hospital)	12.0	15.0	9.5	10.5	11.0	11.0
MRI (freestanding)	0.0	0.0	8.5	9.5	10.0	10.5
Total (volume per day)	12.0	15.0	18.0	20.0	21.0	21.5
Volume per Year						
MRI (hospital)	3,120.0	3,900.0	2,470.0	2,730.0	2,866.5	2,866.5
MRI (freestanding)	0.0	0.0	2,210.0	2,470.0	2,600.0	2,730.0
Total (volume per year)	3,120.0	3,900.0	4,680.0	5,200.0	5,466.5	5,596.5
Net Revenue per Year						
Based on wholesale charge						
MRI (hospital)	$300.00	$1,170,000	$ 741,000	$ 819,000	$ 859,950	$ 859,950
Based on average partnership revenue per procedure						
MRI (freestanding)	$489.23	0	1,081,204	1,208,404	1,272,005	1,335,605
Total (net revenue)		$1,170,000	$1,822,204	$2,027,404	$2,131,955	$2,195,555

to participate, but the ventures have to be under my control and must be available to all members of the medical staff."

Dr. Dalton was somewhat overwhelmed. "Mr. Dealer, I'm right in the middle of office hours now. I really don't have the time to talk. The radiologist is coming into town to set up an MRI center. We've looked at his credentials, his experience, and his previous performance, and he's a legitimate expert. He also appears to know how to run a business, and that will be a significant enhancement to the radiology capabilities in our area. There is no one locally who even approaches his expertise on MRI. It was his desire to work only with the doctors and not have hospital involvement at all. He's been working that way successfully for years. I have spent the last several months convincing him that it would be appropriate to try to do a joint venture with the hospital and physicians. An experienced firm has been hired to structure the joint venture, the same firm that recently completed the cardiac catheterization joint venture with the hospital. The deal is much more favorable to the hospital than it even needs to be. It was my intention that as soon as we had something concrete on paper, I would call you to schedule a meeting and see if a venture could be accomplished. It is my feeling that this venture might bring together the medical staff and the hospital and help with some of the bonding that you have spoken about. I will contact you just as soon as we have things down on paper, and we can meet and discuss the matter further. I'd better get back to my patients now."

"Dalton, I am really disappointed you didn't come to me sooner when this guy first came into town and approached you. We certainly don't need more radiologists in town and we don't need doctors doing joint ventures and then informing the hospital about them. Let's set up an appointment as soon as possible."

"OK, Mr. Dealer, we'll do that."

The meeting that followed involved Mr. Dealer, two of his fiscal analysts, Dr. Dalton, and Dr. Ralph Jacobson, the new MRI specialist. Also present was Mr. Cameron, president of National Resource Management, the firm hired to set up the joint venture.

Mr. Cameron presented the joint venture proposal in detail. The hospital's inpatient MRI unit (a two-year-old GE 1.5 Tesla unit) would be the hospital's contribution to the partnership. This unit would be purchased by the partnership for $1.8 million, and the hospital would use $750,000 of that to purchase 50 percent of the limited partner shares. The difference would be paid back in cash to the hospital when the loan for the project was obtained. In essence, the partnership would be leasing the hospital-based MRI scanner for a cost of $300 per procedure. The hospital would bill and collect its revenue from patients as was customary, and any additional revenues collected over the $300 would be theirs to keep. The outpatient unit would be managed separately, and all expenses, management, and administration of the outpatient unit, as well as the radiologist's fees, would be paid from the revenue collected. After all expenses and fees, projections showed a conservative return averaging between 21 percent and 26 percent for the first five years and averaging 36 percent per year for the first ten years. There would be no additional expenses to the hospital in terms of capital outlay now or in the future.

After the presentation by Mr. Cameron, there was some discussion among the participants, and Mr. Dealer's fiscal analysts chose to reserve comment until they had reviewed the numbers. They did remark that it seemed, at least on the surface, to be a feasible plan. Since the partnership proposal was for two general partners, the hospital and the physician ancillary group, Mr. Dealer stated that he felt there might be some objection from the rest of the medical staff, and he was sure there would be major objections from the radiologists.

Dr. Dalton felt that since all the medical staff were going to be invited to participate in this venture, there should be no major problem with regard to the physician ancillary services being one general partner. He also commented that the radiologists would be able to buy shares in the venture and would be able to continue to do all the hospital work and any outpatient services that physicians chose to send them. In fact, it would encourage them to improve the quality and timeliness of their service, because all physicians, whether they had an investment or not, could now send their cases to either of the facilities. There would be no great harm to the hospital, which would profit from either site, and it would make no difference at all to the investors. The only physicians who would be affected would be those interpreting the films for their professional fees. Therefore, competition would be based on quality and service rather than other factors.

There was a flurry of activity for the next several days. The radiologists were quite vocal in their opposition to the hospital's participation in this venture. Mr. Dealer met with them and was told in no uncertain terms that the hospital should not get involved in this joint venture, but that if the hospital desired, they should create a joint venture with the existing MRI and perhaps put up a new unit themselves and sell this to the medical staff. Dealer himself was not happy about this new fellow coming into town, so he had discussions with the resource management firm regarding doing the joint venture with the hospital radiologists and the hospital, and not involving Dr. Jacobson. Mr. Dealer did talk with the radiologists about incorporating Dr. Jacobson into their group. Two years earlier they had had no interest in hiring him when Dr. Jacobson had called the chief of their section to discuss the possibility of joining their group. Now they were interested in at least talking with him. This message was communicated to Dr. Jacobson, who had already spoken with Dr. Martin, the head of the radiologists.

Dr. Jacobson felt that what he brought to the table was a high level of expertise and excellence in service. He wanted to duplicate the facility that he had set up in his previous location, and rotating physicians to read MRIs just wouldn't be the same. He also had no desire to return to doing general radiology and to taking night call, which he had not done in years. However, he was available to do MRIs at any time should an emergency arise, and he expected to be called by physicians to do studies in the evenings and on weekends. Mr. Dealer spoke with Dr. Jacobson about joining the group, but Dr. Jacobson felt that this most likely could not be worked out. He was simply unwilling to do general radiology and take general radiology night call, and was unwilling to have radiologists without expertise rotating through his outpatient unit to interpret MRIs. He would certainly allow the one or two radiologists trained in MRI to use the outpatient facility, and he expressed eagerness about setting up an educational program for the radiologists and other medical staff with regard to MRI.

The National Resource Management people discussed with Dr. Dalton and his colleagues the possibility of switching and setting up the venture with the hospital and the hospital radiologists, leaving Dr. Jacobson to his own devices. The physicians were not willing to do this, however, because they felt that the hospital MRI service as currently offered was inadequate and was actually the reason for the need for the project. The project would represent the only way of ensuring improved MRI service. The physicians felt that MRI had become too important to the current state-of-the-art practice of several specialties, such as neurology and neurosurgery, orthopedics, and oncology, to allow continuation of the current inadequate service. They felt that the hospital had used its monopoly status to offer poor service, knowing they would get all the business anyway.

Mr. Dealer also had several meetings with his fiscal analysts. Next, a large open meeting was scheduled to present the offer to the medical staff. Selected board members as well as the administration were invited. This meeting took place, and the medical staff expressed a strong interest in pursuing the project. Many medical staff members at the meeting seemed quite happy that the venture did appear to work in the interest of everyone, including the hospital, the physicians, and the consumers. Following the solicitation meeting, Mr. Dealer met again with radiology and with his fiscal analysts. The venture made sense financially and probably could be negotiated for even further hospital advantage, but the outpatient MRI scanner would be under the control of the physician group. There would be the problem of dealing with the hospital radiologists, but they could be offered conditions that would protect their income from being adversely affected for the next two or three years. The venture did not fit well with Mr. Dealer's plan for one grand joint venture involving multiple services, involving the entire medical staff, and with total control in the hands of the hospital management team. However, he was led to believe, by Dr. Jacobson and by the National Resource Management team, that if the hospital did not participate, the joint venture would be restructured to include physicians, the Resource Management team, and Dr. Jacobson, and the hospital would be excluded.

Mr. Dealer knew he had to make a presentation with recommendations to the board the following Tuesday morning. He knew the direction he should take and he called another meeting with his fiscal management team.

Part **IV**

Organizational Design

Commentary

Does Organizational Design Really Matter?

J. Richard Gaintner, M.D.

In his classic text, *Management: Tasks, Practices, and Responsibilities*, Peter F. Drucker says the following about organization design:

> We have learned that organization does not start with structure but with building blocks; that there is no one right or universal design but that each enterprise needs to design around the key activities appropriate to its mission and its strategies; that three different kinds of work—operating, innovative and top-management—require being structured and lodged under the same organizational roof; and that organizational structure needs to be both task-focused and person-focused and to have both an authority axis and a responsibility axis.[1]

The cases that follow illustrate Drucker's points very nicely. Emrich, for example, discusses organizational alternatives in a traditionally and functionally designed department of medicine to facilitate care, education, and research. The department, of course, is also part of a hospital and a medical school in an academic health science center. The case highlights issues such as central versus delegated control, physician autonomy versus "managed" groups, and the all too common dilemma of dollars driving structure and function.

The Johns Hopkins Experiment

The experiment with decentralized management that has occurred at Johns Hopkins Hospital over the last two decades also serves as an excellent illustration of the potential impact of organizational design.[2] In the early 1970s, the hospital's clinical departments (medicine, surgery, and so on) were reorganized into functional units with physician chiefs as the directors (chief executives) of the component "businesses." These physician executives also chair the academic departments in the Johns Hopkins University School of Medicine. An administrator and a nursing director report to each physician "functional unit director." Each unit also has its own financial officer reporting directly to the administrator. Central hospital management has held these units accountable through extensive management and financial information systems with data shared openly among units, with central management, and with the board. The impetus for the new system was the belief that since the chiefs already controlled the use of resources, they should also be accountable for expenditures. Peer pressure among departments was found to more effectively control expenditure excesses than management jawboning. There were financial and other rewards (e.g., more house staff slots) built into the system for performance that was better than anticipated.

The governance, structure, and management of this performance-based system have worked very well for Johns Hopkins, but this is not to suggest that the decentralization approach is right for other institutions. Rather, the important points are these: First, basic organizational design concepts were applied in a complex health care setting with players who were committed to success and excellence. Second, exceptional leadership talent was present in the effort. By looking at the way these features affected the organization's management and operations, we can see the significance of the design and its implementation. In *Creating New Health Care Ventures: The Role of Management*, Regina Herzlinger of the Harvard Business School discusses seven key management functions that are necessary for successful organizations: (1) management control (i.e., accounting), (2) finance, (3) marketing, (4) human resource management, (5) operations management, (6) management of regulation, and (7) clear management philosophy.[3] With the exception of marketing, each of these management functions clearly was present from the outset of the Johns Hopkins decentralized management experiment. Among the most important of these factors were a clear-cut sense of direction built on the foundation of a strong tradition of excellence, very good information systems with broad sharing of the data, and precise accountability lines. Data allowed the functional units to verify monthly performance and allowed central management and the board to hold the units accountable.

Global institutional budgeting and finance were conducted in co-operation with the units, focusing particularly on volume projections from each unit. Once determined, expenditures were totally decentralized. Operating and capital budget requests were presented annually by the departments to central management. Departmental performance was compared internally and data also were compared to those of other similar institutions and to the Maryland rate commission regulations. Capital budgets were prepared by a committee of chiefs, managers, and nurses from central management and the functional units. Central management made final budget recommendations to a joint board-management committee, which then went to the full board. Chiefs attended all board meetings and were granted the privilege of speaking but not voting. Physicians, nurses, managers, and financial people were involved together in every step along the way.

Central administration dealt extensively with regulations. The chief financial officer was especially adept at working with the state and federal regulators. Because of the state-imposed reimbursement system, revenue was not decentralized. Significant financial winners (e.g., oncology) and losers (e.g., pediatrics) were not necessarily related to performance.

There was a central human resources department for policy matters and union negotiations (service and maintenance workers only; not nursing, technical, secretarial, or other categories). Nurses were recruited by central nursing in conjunction with human resources and the decentralized nursing units. Operations were controlled completely by the units that negotiated service arrangements with the central departments. They could seek better prices and services outside the institution, although that rarely happened.

The physician managers of the functional units took a hands-on or hands-off approach, depending upon what was needed. Most placed great confidence in their nonphysician administrators and financial officers, and all relied virtually completely on their nursing directors for managing unit nursing activities. The central vice president for nursing became the professional and executive management role model and probably exercised more actual control than would the traditional nursing vice president with no scheduling and other responsibilities.

Regardless of how they chose to exercise their role, the physician managers were key to the success at Johns Hopkins.[4] They brought to the table their academic and professional credibility, a great willingness to work with each other and their management, nursing, and financial colleagues, and a desire for and pursuit of excellence. Management at Johns Hopkins moved closer to patients—where it should be! There were and continue to be "glitches" in the system, but this organizational design works extremely well in this setting and is one model worthy of serious consideration in this most difficult health care industry.

The Basics behind the Design

Although no one system, style, approach, or philosophy is effective in all places at all times, the basics are still basic! Value, values, and leadership, along with the application of fundamental management principles, are key in any organizational design. In addition, open communication (especially listening) and clear lines of authority, responsibility, and accountability are essential. These factors allow for adaptation to the uniqueness of each setting and time.

Value can be represented by the simple equation $V = Q/C \times E$, where Q represents quality, E represents efficacy, and C represents cost. *Quality* should be measured in terms of the scientific and technical aspects of what is done, along with the degree of humaneness on the part of the doers.[5] The patient's perception of the latter is very important, and for better or worse, this is how he or she really judges quality. Such is the science and art of medicine! *Efficacy* refers to the appropriateness or effectiveness of what is done. David Eddy and others have done much to focus our attention on this parameter.[6] Businesses of the future will not pay for operations or procedures that are not efficacious. After all, if efficacy is rated as zero (i.e., the procedure did not benefit the patient), then the value will always be zero, even if the procedure is done well, artfully, and at low cost! Obviously, the lower the cost, the higher the value, assuming the same level of quality.

Without a set of basic *values* incorporated into a strong management philosophy, the risk of organizational failure is increased. Integrity, the pursuit of excellence, compassion, and other basic human values are essential for the long-term process of any enterprise. Watergate, the Iran-Contra scandal, junk bonds, and the savings and loan crisis are but a few examples of how the absence of basic values leads to a decline in credibility and a loss of accountability.

Leadership is "getting out in front" and providing the kind of direction that people can and will follow. After all, it is the followers who confer leadership status on the individual who attempts to lead. People desire direction and will follow it as long as they have the opportunity to know the direction and to receive regular input and feedback.

Hence, the need for open and frequent communication and effective information systems.

Excellent management and financial information systems are necessary conditions for success, and excellent clinical information systems also are desired. Although fully functional combinations of these information systems are unusual, there is much hope for the future. More patient-centered, on-line systems are under development and testing.

Finally, all this change requires teamwork under any circumstances, especially in the health care environment! Doctors, nurses, managers, and all others must have opportunities to learn to work together, not just for success but for survival. Teamwork is better for patients, too, and is certainly more fun!

At a recent annual meeting of the American College of Physician Executives, Regina Herzlinger noted that physician managers are essential to future success in the health marketplace. She reported that at the Harvard Business School only health care and real estate warrant special "industry" courses. A knowledge of the basic business (caring for sick people) is an essential but insufficient condition for the management of organizations that deal with patients. Physicians seem more amenable to being managed by other physicians than by nonphysician managers. Like it or not, doctors drive the system: admissions, discharges, tests and drugs, operations, and so on. But they also are entrepreneurs and they want autonomy. It is through the careful balancing of autonomy and control, using appropriate mechanisms for accountability, that the desired ends can be achieved.

I am convinced—and have been for the 20-plus years I have been a physician manager—that teams of physicians, nurses, administrators, finance people, marketers, and others can make very beautiful music together! Whether the conductor is a physician or not, harmony must prevail; hence the need for management and leadership. Physician managers are in an excellent position to provide such leadership and be effective conductors so that organizations will create beautiful music!

The Part IV Cases

Physician executives must be concerned with how the work is organized in their own organizations, both before and after their organization merges with another. Organizational structure is important to the stakeholders of health care organizations, who see it vitally affecting their political power, autonomy, and mission.

The cases in Part IV give the reader excellent examples of how organizational design will vary from setting to setting and suggest that there is rarely only one answer or approach, although some organizations are in better shape than others depending on time, place, people, resources, and outside forces. The cases make it clear that physician managers play a vital role today and will continue to do so in the future.

In each of these cases, the way services are organized makes a great deal of difference to the respective academic internists, chiefs of departments, and medical group partners. One consideration is what structure will work best for patient care, research, and teaching. A second is what structure makes sense for the financial viability of the organization. A third is what structure works best for the principal practicing physicians involved. The job of the physician executive is to focus key stakeholders on the organization's mission and to develop solutions that make sense to those paying for service and providing the service. This is no easy accomplishment! In addition to opportunity, there is often a great deal of risk associated with structuring and restructuring decisions—risk for the organization and for the physician executive involved in planning and implementation.

Alternative organizational structures for the department of medicine

Faced with the challenges of a competitive health care market and organizational changes within the university, Dr. Oliver Reynolds thought it was time to look at the structure of his own department. He hired a management consultant who offered three alternatives. When selecting an alternative, he needed to take many issues into consideration. Not only were there structural issues, but whatever he decided would have financial and political effects both on his department and on the university. Was he willing to take the risk of upsetting the status quo? Would it be worth the effort as well as the headaches?

Case questions

1. Why was the current organizational structure adopted?
2. What are the opportunities and threats that affect consideration of alternative organizational structures?
3. What are the advantages and disadvantages of the three alternatives?
4. What do you recommend to Dr. Reynolds? Why?
5. Are there any other options that should be considered? Why or why not?

Merger of the perinatal departments at Morningside Hospital

Planning a merger may seem like an extremely difficult task. It is. Implementing a merger is monumental. The merging of the perinatal departments was just the beginning of the merging process at Morningside. It was important, therefore, that it be well-thought-out and done correctly.

Coming into the merger, the perinatal departments at both Lutheran and Wilkinson had their own identities. The health professionals who worked in each department were immersed in those identities. Trying to merge the two philosophies was like trying to merge the Republican and Democratic parties. Was it possible?

How does a new entity gain its own philosophy? Dr. Boswell decided to plan a staff retreat to work out a solution that would be acceptable to everyone. He knew that a consensus would be necessary in order for the board of directors to accept the recommendation.

This case raises questions about consumer input, marketing, self-determination, well care versus sick care, innovation and creativity, and how to design an organization to achieve maximum value.

Case questions

1. Why isn't Morningside Hospital further advanced in reorganizing obstetrical services by the end of 1987?

2. What could Dr. Boswell have done prior to the merger to avoid the current problems?

3. Who should be invited to the retreat? Who should chair the meeting?

4. What does the market in Bakerville really want?

5. Is the merger of the perinatal departments at Lutheran Hospital and Wilkinson Hospital a sound idea?

6. Which should be the driving force, the financial analysis or the mission?

7. Could there be a successful transition requiring little interruption of care to parents and newborns would occur and little threat to overall quality?

8. Formulate an implementation plan and time line to accomplish all of Morningside's goals.

Governance at Lonetree and Prairie group practices

In a rapidly changing competitive medical environment, two very different group practices find themselves pressured to talk to one another about a possible formal merger. Everyone agrees that the merger would be strategically beneficial but operationally very difficult. They are faced with ownership, management, and governance issues for both their groups and their HMOs.

As in most mergers, each party brings its own history, mission, practice style, and identity. Ironing out these major areas is no small task. This all causes confusion in the community at large, confusion to both sets of employers and even to each practitioner. Sometimes mergers are pushed along by fierce competitive pressures, and the parties are dragged along in the process, kicking and screaming every step of the way.

The case eventually focuses on governance. How can two very different entities govern in a style that is mutually acceptable to everyone and does not compromise their standards?

Case questions

1. Why would a merger of the two medical groups be strategically beneficial?
2. Why would a merger of the two medical groups be operationally very difficult?
3. What would be your idea of fair representation of both groups on the board of directors?
4. Should the CEOs be on the Board? Why or why not?
5. Should everyone have voting rights?
6. Should the members be appointed or elected? By whom?
7. When should terms on the board begin and end?
8. What other issues need to be considered when setting up the governance of a group or institution?

Notes

1. P. F. Drucker, *Management Tasks, Responsibilities, Practices* (New York: Harper and Row, 1973), 517.
2. R. M. Heyssel, J. R. Gaintner, I. W. Kues, A. A. Jones, and S. A. Lipstein. "Decentralized Management in a Teaching Hospital," *New England Journal of Medicine*, 310 (1984): 1477–80.

3. R. Herzlinger, *Creating New Health Care Venture: The Role of Management* (Rockville, MD: Aspen Publishers, 1992). Dr. Herzlinger discussed these points at the ACPE meeting, San Antonio, May 1990.
4. This has also been true in other settings, such as the Harvard teaching hospitals.
5. At the New England Deaconess Hospital in Boston, our mission statement says that we are "a place where science and kindliness unite in combatting disease." This can be attributed to Mary E. Lunn, founding Deaconess, 1896.
6. D. M. Eddy. "The Challenge," *Journal of the American Medical Association*, 263 (1990): 287–90.

Alternative Organizational Structures for the Department of Medicine

James S. Emrich

Stuart James is a senior consultant in the management services division of a major accounting firm. His company has been retained by Dr. Oliver Reynolds, who is the chairman of the Department of Medicine at Ivy Medical School. His assignment is to develop a series of alternative organizational structures and ultimately to recommend a preferred approach, one that will serve the future management needs of the department.

In preparation for undertaking this assignment, James has done some research concerning the evolution of the Department of Medicine and Ivy Medical School during the 1970s and 1980s, as this was a time of turbulent change in the areas of biomedical research, the practice of medicine, and professional instruction and training.

Ivy Medical School continues to be viewed as one of the preeminent medical institutions in the country. Under the leadership of Dr. Thomas Masterman, who succeeded Dean Merriwell, the research base of the medical school has been invigorated to the point where the school now stands among the top five in the country. In

Reprinted from *Health Services Management: A Book of Cases*, 3d ed., edited by A. R. Kovner and D. Neuhauser, 82–104 (Ann Arbor, MI: Health Administration Press, 1989), with permission, Health Administration Press.

addition, Dean Masterman foresaw the increasingly important role clinical practice would play in funding schools of medicine, and therefore pioneered the development of one of the nation's first faculty practice plan organizations spanning multiple departments within the school.

Another important organizational development involves the creation of a medical center management and governance function. Historically, Ivy Medical School and Ivy University Hospital were overseen by independent executives who, in turn, reported to a common vice president within the university. This vice president had responsibility for all health science activities, including the schools of dentistry, allied medical professions, and nursing, in addition to medicine and the university hospital. Recently, the president of the university decided to create an academic medical center composed of the school, the university hospital, and the faculty practice plan. He established the role of executive vice president of the medical center, directly accountable to himself. He also requested that the university trustees create a governance mechanism that would provide the appropriate fiduciary oversight of medical center activities.

Within a relatively short period of time, Dr. Ivan Markham resigned as chairman of medicine to assume a senior position in the Public Health Service in the United States Department of Health and Human Services. After a lengthy search, the chair was assumed by Dr. Reynolds, an oncologist of international repute, who had been chairman of medicine in two other schools previously. Although formerly a very productive researcher with a modest clinical practice, upon assuming the chair at Ivy, Dr. Reynolds concentrated on the management and administration of his department.

Upon his arrival, Dr. Reynolds was confronted with a department that was deeply in debt. Overall research productivity was low, as measured by the level of National Institutes of Health (NIH) peer review funding, and the department's clinical capacity was significantly underutilized. Ivy Hospital's occupancy problems continued to deteriorate and there was extreme pressure on Dr. Reynolds to fill beds.

Over the course of the next several years, Dr. Reynolds was able to meet the challenges placed before him. He doubled the number of faculty members, including many full-time clinicians, and thus managed to increase significantly the level of ambulatory and inpatient activity. Both case and patient-day levels rose by more than 30 percent, to the point where the Department of Medicine consistently exceeded its available complement of beds at Ivy Hospital. Given the prevailing fee-for-service method of physical payment, the department benefited financially from these initiatives. Over the course of one decade, the

Department of Medicine was transformed from one of the poorest departments to the most financially robust.

The above successes notwithstanding, Dr. Reynolds has recently become uneasy about what the future holds for his department. As a result, he has hired Mr. James, whose firm also serves as the auditor for Ivy University.

The Assignment

Dr. Reynolds's initial interview with Mr. James went as follows:

REYNOLDS: Stuart, by any measure of performance, this department has been very successful over the last decade. We have renewed our faculty by bringing on competent young researchers and clinicians. We have taken a leadership role in revising and implementing the clinical curriculum for medical students and have increased the size of our departmental graduate and postgraduate training programs to more than 200 persons per year. Our clinical practice grew significantly in the early 1980s and still grows at a reasonable rate, and we fill our beds in the hospital and then some. As a result of this, we are financially very sound.

I am concerned, however, about what the future holds for us. In the area of research, the level of NIH funding in constant dollars is essentially static. Yet the competition for these funds has increased significantly as a result of an increased number of academic physicians being trained by our nation's medical schools. I also perceive threats on the clinical practice front, as there is increasing competition among hospitals and physicians in this area as institutions fight for *market share.* That, by the way, is a term I never thought I would hear myself utter! Taking this all into account, I believe we may be entering an era of limited resources as we exit a decade of sustained growth. In light of this, my gut tells me that the organizational structure of the department needs to be rethought. That is why you are here.

Before we examine the current organizational structure, I would like to share with you what has been my approach to the management of this department. To put it bluntly, the overriding factor influencing my management style was that we were broke. Accordingly, when I arrived, I put strong financial controls in, which essentially made it impossible for any significant amount of money to be spent without my prior approval. I am sure this was seen by many as a harsh action, but I believed it to be absolutely essential in order to restore fiscal solvency.

I immediately encouraged Phil Blue, who was business manager for our research and teaching programs, to seek opportunities elsewhere and hired myself a tough, smart controller. Nancy Sanders assumed this post some nine years ago. She has two principal attributes. First, she is absolutely loyal to me, and second, she knows how and where every dollar is spent.

On the practice side, Ben Goldsmith, who was hired by my predecessor, has been with us for almost 15 years. He is a very capable administrator who has developed a high level of expertise in physician billing. Ben, too, is very loyal to both the department and me, although I must confess that my interaction with him is limited by the pressures on my time. Besides, as my father always used to say, "If it ain't broke, don't fix it!"

Ben and Nancy, then, are the two key lay managers in our department. In addition, I have appointed two members of our faculty to serve in the part-time roles of leading our residency program and overseeing our responsibilities for providing clinical instruction to medical students.

JAMES: Excuse me, Dr. Reynolds, but it seems to me what you are describing is like a wheel with a hub and spokes—and you are the hub. How can you possibly keep up with, much less actively manage, this myriad of activities?

REYNOLDS: That's precisely the point. I cannot, and I am not alone. This is the dilemma that most of my peers face in other departments of medicine across the country. Like me, many of them have, with real regret, given up any active involvement in research and seeing private patients. For many years now, I have been a full-time manager, something I never contemplated when I entered medical school.

Let me show you, then, the organizational charts of the medical center and our department. (See Figures 10.1 and 10.2.) As you can see, within the department, essentially all functions report directly to me. I should also point out that insofar as the medical center is concerned, I am accountable to the school for my conduct as chairman, to the hospital for managing our inpatient service and directing a series of complex diagnostic and therapeutic programs, and to my fellow chairs in the faculty practice plan inasmuch as the Department of Medicine provides a significant number of referrals to these other departments.

Given all of this, Stuart, how are you going to approach this analysis?

JAMES: Well, the one thing that is very clear to me is that you have multiple constituencies. While this is true of any chief executive—and that, by the way, is what you are—of any organization of even modest

Figure 10.1   The Medical Center at Ivy University

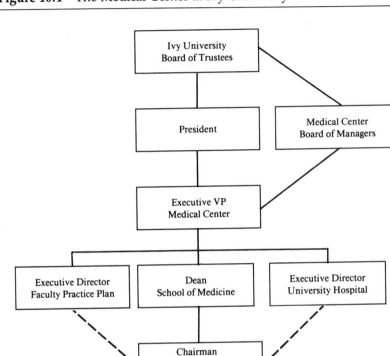

size, it seems to me that your situation is even more complex than what one would find in industry. Thus, while there are some basic organizational principles that I am sure I can apply to your situation, it is particularly important to me to get varied perspectives of your departmental enterprise. Therefore, I plan to conduct a series of interviews with several people within your department. These would include a section chief, a busy clinical faculty member, Nancy Sanders, and Ben Goldsmith. I would also like to meet with the senior business executive of the school of medicine, to ascertain his views on this important issue.

Once I have completed my interviews, I will return to you with some organizational options, although I must stress right now that while I may have a preference for one or the other, what is most important is that you are comfortable with the proposed solution.

Figure 10.2   The Department of Medicine at Ivy Medical School: Current

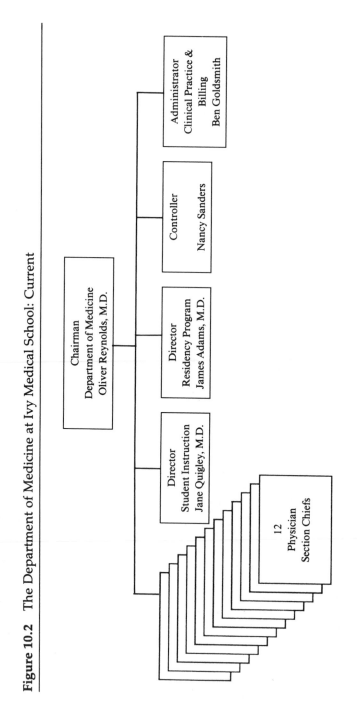

Dr. Richard Thomas

Mr. James then proceeded to conduct a series of five fact-finding interviews with the various individuals whom he and Dr. Reynolds had agreed upon.

The first interview was with Dr. Richard Thomas, the chief of the rheumatology section. Dr. Thomas is a solid scientist with an active clinical practice and an excellent regional reputation as an expert in arthritis. He has been chief of the section for more than 20 years and has been on the faculty at Ivy University since his fellowship almost 35 years ago. As he is wont to say, "I have seen deans and chairmen come and go!" Dr. Thomas, who is the most senior of the section chiefs, was selected for interview by Dr. Reynolds because his opinion will be an important one to consider with respect to any possible reorganization.

JAMES: As you know, Dr. Thomas, my firm has been retained by Dr. Reynolds to assess the current organizational structure of the Department of Medicine with an eye toward what will be necessary in the years to come. With this in mind, I would appreciate it if you would give me your views on the current strengths and weaknesses of the department and how, if at all, organizational improvements might be made.

THOMAS: Well, Mr. James, first let me begin by saying that I have great respect for what the chairman has been able to accomplish during the last decade. In particular, he has restored the financial health of this department, and I am hopeful that the funds we have collectively been able to accumulate will now be used to invest in the future. We have a crying need for more research space, and our clinical practice activity is also becoming increasingly crowded. More than anything, we need room to grow.

Oliver did call me a few days ago to brief me on the reasons for this interview. Frankly, I believe this management business is highly overrated. First, we physicians are a very independent group, who, as professionals, value autonomy highly. We are also among the intellectual elite of our society, having been trained to ask important questions and solve difficult problems based not only upon hard data but also upon clinical and scientific judgment.

Please don't misunderstand me. I certainly believe that we need competent administration. Someone surely needs to order the supplies and keep the books. In fact, my administrative assistant, Betsy, is a perfect example of this. She started with me some 25 years ago as a clerk typist and has worked her way up through the ranks to her current position. During this time, she has learned the techniques of office management from a practical standpoint, and she has also taken a few accounting courses at night. She keeps me out of trouble and lets me know everything that is going on, and I do mean everything! In my opinion, the real problem that Oliver has is that he does not have someone like Betsy in his office.

JAMES: Dr. Thomas, these are very important observations, but don't you think that given the unsettled times in your field some sort of organizational change might be advisable?

THOMAS: I am afraid, Mr. James, that you are still not getting my point. The members of our faculty pride themselves on their ability to make an individual contribution to our missions of advancing the frontiers of knowledge, transmitting our current knowledge to those receiving instruction, and providing patient service. We do so in a very personal way. In the laboratory, we are the principal investigators. In the classroom, we are the professors. In the clinics and wards, we are the respected physicians. In truth, while Ivy University has a great tradition, its reputation in the eyes of the public is no more than the sum of the reputations of the individual faculty members.

However, before we close our interview, I would like to comment upon a couple of other points with respect to our current state of affairs. First, the chairman has much too tight a hold on our departmental purse strings. In the old days, I was able to spend pretty much as I pleased, although, mind you, I knew that I had to make ends meet in the long run. Now, it seems that I am in the chairman's office every time I want to spend even $50,000 or so. Even smaller scale expenditures are closely watched. Nancy Sanders is constantly questioning me about one financial transaction or another. I am not used to this kind of treatment, and quite frankly, I don't care much for it. I also know that several other chiefs feel similarly.

One final point I would like to make is that the chairman does not consult with his section chiefs on a regular enough basis. To be sure, we have extensive discussions about any matter that is of direct impact on an individual section. What I am talking about here are policy issues that are of importance to the entire department. I truly believe that we would have a clearer sense of where we are going and how we might get there if there were some mechanism for meeting as a group with the chairman on a regular basis.

JAMES: Tell me, if you would, how you accomplish this within your own section.

THOMAS: I don't, because it simply isn't necessary. We number only 15 faculty members in all and are fortunate enough to have our research space and clinical space in contiguous areas. Communication is, therefore, excellent albeit informal. Besides, I make it a point to tell my faculty members whatever they need to know.

As you can tell by now, Mr. James, I am very skeptical about the worth of your endeavor. However, I do hope I will see some of my suggestions incorporated into your final proposal. You may wish to get back to me so that I might review some of your ideas in draft form.

Dr. Ralph Watson

Next no Mr. James's interview list is Dr. Ralph Watson, the chief of cardiology. Dr. Watson is 45 years old and assumed his post approximately five years ago. He was trained as an interventional cardiologist and still carries a modest caseload. He was selected by Dr. Reynolds because he is representative of the "new generation" of academic physicians and because of the obvious influence that sections of cardiology have on departments of medicine.

JAMES: Dr. Watson, I appreciate your taking time out of your busy day to review with me some of the important issues facing the Department of Medicine in the future. I believe Dr. Reynolds has spoken with you about the basic objectives of my consulting engagement.

WATSON: Yes. Ollie did talk to me briefly and I certainly agree we need to do something. This department has simply gotten too big and unwieldy. What's more, I am afraid that we are overemphasizing basic research, that is, the cellular and molecular level. While I would be the first to admit that discoveries of incalculable worth are being made as a result of the application of techniques of this "new" science, we in the clinical departments should be focusing our attention on research using animal models, on clinical research, and most especially on patients. After all, that is what we have ultimately been trained to do, to take care of patients! While I acknowledge this is a research university, we are doctors and there should be much more emphasis on clinical medicine.

I already alluded to what I think is the main problem when I noted our excessive size and diversity. Over the course of the last two to three decades, we have become a much more heterogeneous discipline. For decades, the trademark of a specialist in internal medicine was his or her ability to diagnose a disease. Resulting therapeutic intervention, whether with drugs or involving surgery, was relatively straightforward. Often, this would involve a referral to some other specialist. The last 30 years, however, have seen an enormous increase in interventional internal medicine. By this I mean that we have expanded our capability to diagnose and to intervene therapeutically, particularly in organ systems built around pulmonary medicine, gastrointestinal medicine, and cardiology. The most extreme example of this is in cardiology, where we are now essentially doing procedures that in the past would have been classified as surgical. All of this means we have a much closer relationship with the hospital than even with our own department, not unlike what has historically occurred with radiology, pathology, and anesthesiology.

There is another very important issue at hand here, and that is the one of compensation. While each of us in our section has made a conscious commitment to academic medicine, the compensation differential between this setting and community teaching hospitals has become enormous. Virtually every day the members of my faculty are receiving offers from large community teaching hospitals guaranteeing the doubling or tripling of their salary. You have to be awfully dedicated to continue to ignore those kinds of differences and what they can mean to your lifestyle and that of your family.

Compensation, then, is a key issue to cardiology. In all candor, the chairman's ability to deal with this is limited. I believe this is because he needs to maintain some relative equity of compensation across the entire department, and our section is so unusual that we simply do not fit into any rational scheme. It is a highly skewed situation inasmuch as we produce 45 percent of the department's clinical income and yet receive only 20 percent of the relevant clinical compensation. Put bluntly, the research mission of the department is being carried on the backs of my cardiologists. While this is not entirely new, this imbalance is becoming more and more extreme.

JAMES: Dr. Watson, if I understand you correctly, you are describing a phenomenon that is probably generic to departments of medicine across the country. If so, are there other models for addressing these problems?

WATSON: Yes, the answer is simple but painful. As I said before, cardiology is becoming increasingly like other hospital-based specialties with an equipment-intensive diagnostic and therapeutic approach. Procedure-based medicine has always been much more highly compensated than cognitive medicine, and this is the dilemma we face in the Department of Medicine. My solution is to create a separate and distinct Department of Cardiology.

I now this is a highly controversial suggestion, but to put it in business terms you are used to dealing with, the conglomerate approach to departments of medicine simply is not working. Why, if we would be allowed to, my faculty might even be willing to consider a leveraged buyout.

JAMES: Well, Dr. Watson, you certainly have some striking views on the question of the organization of the department. May I ask you, however, to set aside your self-described, somewhat radical notion and focus on some of the organizational needs of the department, assuming cardiology remains an important constituent part?

WATSON: As you can see, Mr. James, I really do not hold out much hope for maintaining this department as a unified whole. However, if there is any hope, I believe it lies in the creation of a small executive committee to assist the chairman in establishing our future direction. I want to emphasize the notion of small. The chairman needs to gather around him three or four trusted faculty members who have both the vision as to where academic medicine is going and the power to make that vision a reality. This wouldn't be a debating society; it would be an action-oriented group. Of course, the chief of cardiology would have to be a member of such a group.

Excuse me, Mr. James, but I believe our time is up. I have patients waiting.

Ben Goldsmith

The next interview for Mr. James was with Ben Goldsmith, the administrator of the group practice. While taking pride in doing a good job, Ben continues to be relatively satisfied with his current role in the organization. In particular, he is pleased with the balance he has been able to maintain between his personal life and his vocation.

JAMES: Ben, I am looking forward to our discussion about the challenges confronting the Department of Medicine and the potential for future organizational responses to those challenges. As you know, I am conducting a series of interviews in order to give myself as broad a view as possible. So far, I have been focusing on discussions with physician leaders within the department, including Drs. Thomas and Watson. Now it is time for me to turn my attention to the full-time managers in the department. If you wouldn't mind, I would like you to give me a thumbnail sketch of the current level of practice activity.

GOLDSMITH: Our group practice operation has thrived during the 15 years that I have been here. We now have more than 140 physicians who participate in part or in full in delivering clinical services to patients. We provide more than 100,000 ambulatory visits on an annual basis and admit approximately 6,500 patients to the hospital. Our average daily census exceeds 160 patients, even though we have been able to reduce our length of stay by over two days in the last several years. All this translates to an excess of $20 million in collections split approximately equally between inpatient revenue and outpatient revenue. This represents more than a fivefold increase since I first joined the department back in the early 1970s.

JAMES: Ben, I see by reviewing historical department documents that when you came on board, it was proposed that there be developed a group practice advisory committee with a chair who would report directly to the chairman of medicine. Was this structure implemented and, if so, how did it work out?

GOLDSMITH: Yes, that structure was essentially implemented and it has been in place during my entire tour of duty with the Department of Medicine. I did, however, negotiate one important change in that I retained an independent and direct reporting relationship to the chairman of medicine. The group practice committee then became an advocacy group for issues and concerns revolving around the clinical practice of medicine. I meet with this group on a regular basis to receive their suggestions and understand their problems as they relate to the operational support we provide. The chairman of this committee meets with Dr. Reynolds on an ad hoc basis to review policy concerns.

In all candor, this structure has not worked as well as I had hoped. Frankly, I do not know whether it is because of the personalities involved or whether it is a reflection of this particular organizational arrangement or some combination of both. What I do know is that the chairman of the practice advisory committee and I do not seem to be on the same wavelength and that we seem to continue to focus on the details of the practice operation as opposed to where it might be headed. Also, while I understand it, my access to Dr. Reynolds has been very limited over the years. I know that he is a very busy man and I do not take it personally, but I am concerned that there are important clinical practice issues of long-term significance, which are not being brought to his attention in an orderly and thoughtful way.

JAMES: What's missing, Ben? Leaving aside the issue of having a difference in personalities, are there any organizational initiatives that seem important to you?

GOLDSMITH: Yes, I think there are two. First, it is clear to me that I need a strong physician ally who is viewed as part of management. The role of the physician advisory group is not clear. Is it meant to be a form of quasi-self-governance for the clinical faculty, or is it meant to be an advisory group? Is it meant to focus on short-range operational issues, or is it meant to address issues of long-range concern to the clinical practice of medicine? My own view is that this group should be focusing much more on the issues of long-range impact, leaving the operational details to me. This notwithstanding, I am fully aware that we need to keep the clinical perspective clearly in mind as we make day-to-day operational decisions. Thus, I absolutely need a physician colleague, not a committee, who has credibility with the faculty, who will advise me and ultimately support me in my day-to-day decision making.

Now for my other point, which concerns the relationship between my office and the department business office.

JAMES: I am glad you're bringing this up, Ben, since I will be interviewing Nancy Sanders next.

GOLDSMITH: Let me preface my remarks by saying that I have the highest respect for Nancy's professional qualifications as an accountant and for the job that she has done in assisting Dr. Reynolds in restoring the financial health of this department. Certainly, she has served him with the utmost professional fidelity. I must also say that I am more than a little envious of her ability to meet with the chairman seemingly as frequently as she needs to. I assume that this is probably because she is just down the hall from him.

As you might expect, Nancy and I do not always see eye to eye on certain issues, and she has an opinion on most everything, particularly if it involves spending money. This certainly isn't personal, but it does reflect our different organizational responsibilities. The point I am trying to make is that it now falls to the chairman to try to make sense out of whose proposed course of action on a given matter is most appropriate to support. Somehow, some way, it seems to me that we need to reconcile these various differences without involving the chairman.

JAMES: Well, Ben, our time is drawing to a close and I wonder if there is any thing else on your mind that you would like to suggest.

GOLDSMITH: To be honest with you, when Dr. Reynolds announced that you had been retained to conduct this study, there was a good deal of surprise and some apprehension as to what it all meant. In particular, there has been a lot of speculation that my performance here as practice administrator is under review. Is this true?

JAMES: Unfortunately, Ben, simple questions do not always yield simple answers. No, I am not here to review the performance of you or any other member of the department. However, I cannot make recommendations to the chairman about possible organizational alternatives in a vacuum. One simply cannot and should not completely divorce questions of organizational structure from the question of who will occupy the roles in a proposed structure. As far as I know, you have been doing a fine job in your current capacity. But even you have indicated that you need some additional help in the form of a physician colleague, and you have also raised the question of how clinical operations and financial management are integrated. Let me also reassure you that some degree of anxiety is perfectly natural in situations like this and may even be healthy if it results in self-examination concerning managerial behavior. My best advice to you is just to keep on doing a good job!

Nancy Sanders

The next interview was with Nancy Sanders, who serves as controller for the department. Nancy, a certified public accountant, was hired by Dr. Reynolds about two years after his arrival. She succeeded Phil Blue, who retired after 40 years of service with the school of medicine.

JAMES: Nancy, thanks for taking time out of your busy day to see me. I am aware that this is a very hectic time of year for you given that you are in the process of closing the books and working with your auditors.

SANDERS: It's no problem, I am pleased to talk with you. Besides, when Dr. Reynolds says it's important, it's important!

JAMES: I wonder, then, if you might share with me some of your thoughts about the organizational problems confronting the department at this time.

SANDERS: Well, as you know, my official title is Controller. In reality, I am also the chief financial officer. Thus, I have concerns not only about the control of expenses but also the management of assets.

First, let me make clear that academia is unlike any other business you have ever been exposed to. There is a degree of independence of thought and action that most businesses would not, indeed could not, tolerate. Thus, there is very little respect for routine operating procedure, which, as you know, is the heart of a reliable accounting system. Indeed, it often seems to me that individual section chiefs and their respective business administrators go out of their way to find innovative approaches to beating the system. It certainly makes my job challenging and, in fact, is probably one of the reasons that I like it so much. In a sense, it's a battle of wits!

JAMES: Nancy, that certainly is a different perspective and one that would seem to be fairly healthy under the circumstances. Are there any fundamental organizational issues you feel need to be addressed?

SANDERS: Quite definitely, and they relate to the relationship of my financial services division to both the practice administration activity and the business administration activity that take place within the sections of the department.

First, if I may, a comment about patient billing. As you know, Ben Goldsmith is responsible not only for the administration of the clinical practice but also for the patient-billing function. I am told he is quite expert in the latter and I have no reason to dispute this, although I would note that we have an occasional problem in valuing the receivables. In fact, this is my very point. No self-respecting chief financial officer would allow the management of a major asset such as patient receivables to take place out of her immediate purview. Those are *my* financial statements that are prepared on a quarterly basis, and *my* name is on the line in terms of their accuracy. Put quite simply, I do not believe it is appropriate for that function to report any place other than to finance.

My second point has to do with the functions of business administrators in each of our sections. As I am sure you have gathered by now, many of our individual sections are, in and of themselves, quite substantial enterprises. As a result, many of them have their own business administrator and additional staff. This seems to be a needless waste of resources when, with only a modest addition to the staff in our central office, I am sure that we could serve the needs of each and every section. This would also help to ensure a more uniform application of accounting procedures, appropriate acquisition of supplies and equipment, and strict adherence to university policies.

All in all, I guess it would be fair to say that I am strongly in favor of increased centralization of certain key business functions. I think this not only serves to minimize the current unacceptably high level of business risk inherent in our operations, but it also undoubtedly provides for some economies of scale.

JAMES: That's very interesting, Nancy. Over and above the positive benefits that you believe would be obtained from this centralization, do you see this helping Dr. Reynolds in any way?

SANDERS: Definitely. I don't like surprises and neither does Dr. Reynolds. This would serve to reduce the probability of a material adverse surprise. It should also enable us to provide Dr. Reynolds with even more timely and accurate information, so that he can make the appropriate decisions.

I guess this brings us back to where we started. As far as I'm concerned, Dr. Reynolds is the department, and perhaps to a lesser extent the converse is also true. While challenging, it makes life relatively simple. I have only one person to please!

Patrick Johnson

The next interview was with Patrick Johnson, who is the associate dean for business management at Ivy Medical School. He holds a doctorate in educational administration and has been a senior management executive at Ivy Medical School for more than a decade.

JAMES: Dr. Johnson, I have been looking forward to this interview for some time. To date, all the discussions I have had have been with individuals in the department. I feel it is important to refine some of my impressions with the kind of external perspective you can provide. I believe you are well aware of the nature of my assignment, and it would be very helpful to me if you would share with me your impressions on what you feel needs to be done.

JOHNSON: First, let me say that Dr. Reynolds is highly respected in the school and in this medical center. While this would be true of almost any chairman of medicine because of the importance this position plays in the medical school, Dr. Reynolds has brought his own force of character and vision to the position so that you have a very powerful combination of an important position occupied by an influential person.

Now, I would like to reflect with you about the last ten years that I have spent as associate dean. It has been a time of unparalleled growth, in terms of both the size of our organization and its complexity. Up until quite recently, we have not responded to these changes in any formal way. However, with the development of the medical center entity, the possibility exists for a fundamentally new approach to managing this enterprise. Indeed, I believe that decisions about how the medical center is to function materially affect not only the role of the department chairman but also, in some sense, the management programs of each department.

Dean Masterman was appointed as the executive vice president of the medical center about two years ago. Over that period of time, he has recruited a new general director of Ivy Hospital, a new dean of the medical school, and a new administrator of our faculty practice plan. These individuals all have less than one year of experience in their current position, and all are carefully assessing the management needs of their particular business unit. In so doing, I believe they are taking largely a vertical and functional perspective. They seem to be conceptualizing their management needs in terms of the development of central functions. Thus, the hospital is largely concerned with the delivery of institutional services, the faculty practice plan with the delivery of professional physician services, and the school with the delivery of research and instruction.

Now operationally, the way in which these services are delivered is largely through the departmental organization. Thus, we depend upon the department chairs to oversee the organizational initiatives in these three programmatic areas, while at the same time developing their faculty and, by the way, maintaining some semblance of fiscal stability. This is a daunting task, to say the least. What I am trying to highlight for you is that the department chairs serve as the point of integration across the three identifiable business units of the medical center.

JAMES: If that's so, Dr. Johnson, are those chairs prepared to play that role, and do they have adequate support?

JOHNSON: As to your first question, the answer is "certainly," although most often they conceptualize it in terms of their own particular department and less frequently recognize their responsibility to span the boundaries of the school, the practice plan, and the hospital. As to your second question, we have not, at this point in time, provided or encouraged the chairs to recruit the kind of sophisticated management talent that would help them remain self-sufficient and to some extent autonomous at the department level.

While it is an oversimplification, I believe that we are at the point of having to decide whether the principal management focus is within the three operating units and is largely top down, or whether we should be developing high-level operations management capability within each department in support of the chair. Neither approach is per se correct, but I do think we will need to make a choice.

I should add, in passing, that Dr. Reynolds is the first of the chairs to bring in an outside consultant to help him review what his organizational needs are now and what they are likely to be in the future. I view this to be a very positive step and am pleased to have participated in the process. I am sure you understand that the implications of your assessment and recommendations are potentially broader than simply the Department of Medicine.

Dr. Oliver Reynolds

The final interview was between Mr. James and Dr. Reynolds.

JAMES: Dr. Reynolds, I have completed my analysis and am in a position to share with you three alternatives for future organizational design. I would caution you, however, to view these charts as, at best, an abstraction of the very complex management process necessary to support your department. Indeed, organizational relationships in your department would best be displayed along three dimensions: divisional/ sectional management responsibilities, functional management responsibilities, and program management responsibilities. It is very clear, therefore, that for any structure to be truly effective, a number of mediating organizational mechanisms are probably required, including special task forces, advisory groups, and committees formed to look at specific issues and/or solve specific problems.

As I have conducted my interviews and reflected upon them, three major themes have emerged. First is the need for integration. Some have characterized academic enterprises as "organized anarchies," and in many cases this is not far from the truth. For you, the problem is to achieve a greater sense of cohesiveness while still maintaining the relative independence of your section chiefs and faculty. I believe this is best accomplished through a more highly articulated management structure within your department. There is also a clear need for integrating the activities of your department within the context of the overall medical center.

The second important issue is the need for an identifiable clinical management presence. While you are, by title, chief of service at Ivy Hospital, it is clear that you do not have enough time to devote to this function. This affects not only your faculty's perception of your interest in this area but also the degree of direction your administrative manager receives in supporting the clinical practice.

The final area is governance vis-à-vis management. Intuitively, you understand the desire, indeed the requirement, of professionals to govern or regulate themselves. In addition to management questions, then, there also appears to be a deficit in the area of structure for professional self-governance.

Now we come to an important paradox, and that is that the development of greater structure, in the areas of both management and governance, would appear to fly in the face of the desires of your faculty for maximal autonomy. In many ways, this dilemma will be heightened by the fact that the management reorganization suggestions definitely imply a greater concentration of authority and power.

REYNOLDS: Stuart, you are quite right. The faculty and, most particularly, the section chiefs will be quite skeptical of such an arrangement. Is there no way to mitigate this perceived effect?

JAMES: In the short run, probably not directly. In the longer run, if the management programs that result from the revised organizational structure demonstrate that they are truly serving the faculty, then the problems will diminish somewhat. Equally important, if not more so, is the need to develop a stronger governance structure as a counterbalance, in the minds of the faculty, to a more highly articulated management program. Without this, the perception will be that the "business people" are taking over.

With the above in mind, Dr. Reynolds, I would now like to present to you three alternative organizational arrangements. (See Figures 10.3, 10.4, and 10.5.) First, let me say that all three alternatives have a common view of the need for additional governance mechanisms. There-fore, I have recommended the creation of a departmental advisory com-mittee, which would be composed of the 12 section chiefs and various other programmatic and management leaders of the department. While I have characterized this as an advisory body in its initial stages, you may wish to consider whether or not such an entity might evolve to-ward an executive committee with more delegated authority in certain policy areas.

Given this consistent approach to the governance issue in all three alternatives, the differences revolve around the structuring of the role for a new business executive and a clinical services leaders.

Let me draw your attention to Alternative 1, which I characterize as the classic corporate approach. Simply put, the rationale for this chart revolves around developing a chief operating officer role. This person would be the senior operations management executive of the depart-ment and would have reporting to him or her all central business man-agement functions, including finance, personnel, practice management, and billing. Carried to a logical conclusion, this approach would also imply a line relationship between the business managers in the sections and this chief operating officer. Conceptually, this approach is quite straightforward and deceptively simple to implement in that it involves hiring only one person. It has the potential, however, of profoundly changing the power relationships within the department and therefore may be too radical.

Alternative 2 involves the creation of a new physician executive role to oversee the clinical practice of medicine in your department. I would envision this person as serving as the de facto chief of service of the hospital, although you might retain the titular designation. This physician executive is directly accountable for the total operating perfor-mance of the clinical practice activity, and as a result the proposal is to have the administrator report directly to him or her. I have also retained the direct reporting relationship between Nancy Sanders and yourself under this alternative. Nonetheless, it is necessary that there be a greater degree of cohesion between the practice management and bill-ing areas and the financial shop, and it is not reasonable to expect either you or the new clinical services executive to accomplish this. This, then, implies the need for a senior administrator to oversee the central management activities. The problem is, of course, that you are giving someone considerable responsibility without the requisite authority. While I would never make such a proposal in a more traditional man-agement setting, I do believe this option has some merit, particularly if you want to retain your direct relationship with the financial function and if the clinical chief you recruit requires direct oversight of the

Figure 10.3   The Department of Medicine at Ivy Medical School: Proposed (Alternative 1)

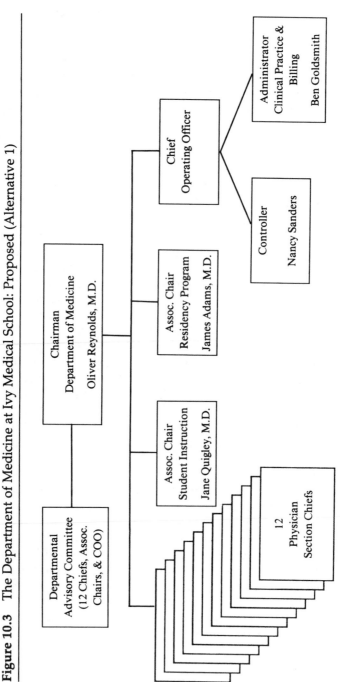

Figure 10.4 The Department of Medicine at Ivy Medical School: Proposed (Alternative 2)

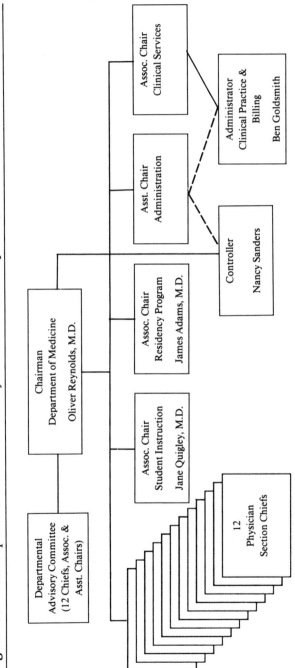

Figure 10.5   The Department of Medicine at Ivy Medical School: Proposed (Alternative 3)

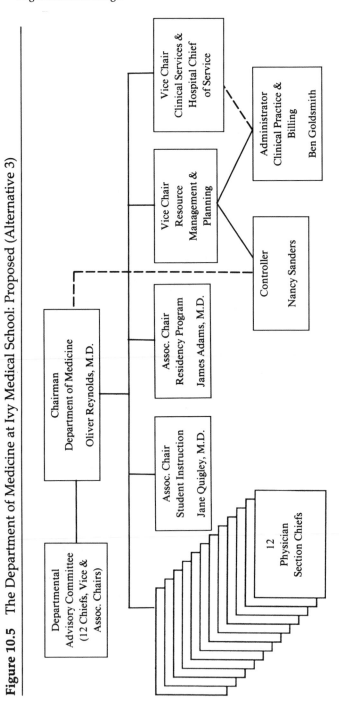

practice operations. I would caution, however, that filling this position will be most difficult. I'm not sure you will get the kind of seasoned executive you will need to take a job designed in this particular way.

Alternative 3 is essentially a combination of the first two in that it combines the notion of a chief operating officer along with the development of a physician executive role in the clinical practices. You will also note that I have changed the title of these two new positions to that of Vice Chair, which is intended to denote that the incumbents in these positions would serve as your two most senior central department executives.

REYNOLDS: Stuart, I thank you for your efforts, although in all candor I am somewhat disappointed by the outcome. It has confirmed my worst fears that there does not appear to be any straightforward management fix to the challenges we are experiencing, although I guess I knew all along that this would be the case. Nonetheless, your analysis has clearly demonstrated that some changes are in order and has increased my resolve to make those changes.

JAMES: May I inquire, Dr. Reynolds, if you are inclined toward any one of the three solutions I have offered?

REYNOLDS: At this point, I really don't know. I'll have to sleep on it. I'll certainly get back to you when I have a clearer indication.

Merger of Perinatal Departments at Morningside Hospital

Scott A. Braucht and Beverly Hills

By mid-June of 1987, five months had passed since the official merger of two multispecialty hospitals located in Bakerville, a metropolitan area with a population of 250,000, located in the south-central region of the United States. The merger of these two facilities, Lutheran Hospital and Wilkinson Hospital, was needed for the financial survival of both. Unfortunately, there were difficult decisions ahead regarding the delivery of all of the clinical services at both hospitals. Although the logistics of the merger had been worked out on paper, the process of building new working relationships among the physicians, clinical staff, and management was in its earliest stage of development. Because of the demand for high-quality, family-centered obstetrical services in the community, and the intense public scrutiny of the effect the hospital merger would have on the area, one of the first issues to be addressed was the consolidation of the perinatal departments within the newly merged institution. Many groups who were watching activities in this area assumed it would not be cost-effective if obstetrical care continued to be provided independently within the two separate facility sites.

Dr. Tim Boswell, the medical director of the newly merged Morningside Hospital, sat at his desk, carefully reviewing general information on maternity programs (Appendix 11.1) and the history of the perinatal programs at both hospital sites. He was reading a few excerpts from a report that discussed marketplace, regulatory, and environmental factors that undoubtedly affected the provision of obstetrical and perinatal services in Bakerville during the mid- to late 1980s.

Morningside's Program

In 1986, prior to the merger, Lutheran Hospital and Wilkinson Hospital held a combined market share of 55.5 percent of the women delivering in Bakerville hospitals. By 1988, the market share of Morningside deliveries was expected to fall to 50 percent, a loss of 5.5 percent in two years, with the delivery base shifting almost entirely to a local Catholic institution, St. Catherine's Hospital. Morningside was showing a decisive loss of market share in the county, as well as in surrounding counties. In addition, there was a concomitant shift in physician referral patterns for tertiary care services, which was having an impact on Morningside's special care nursery admissions and other high-risk obstetrics services. There were a number of reasons for the shift in market share, perhaps the most significant of which was consumer choice. Bakerville Health Cooperative, a staff-model HMO, cited consumer preference as the driving force behind its decision to affiliate with St. Catherine's for normal obstetrical services. Obstetricians at Doctors' Clinic, a large primary care practice in Bakerville, indicated that while they preferred to practice at Wilkinson Hospital, their patients were actively choosing delivery at St. Catherine's.

The most dramatic shift in market share occurred in 1987. In March of that year, St. Catherine's opened its Birthday Suites, a newly renovated facility supporting the labor, delivery, and recovery (LDR) system of obstetrical care. The facility operated with a strong sense of purpose and a solid identity based on a well-written and well-communicated mission statement. Within six months, St. Catherine's experienced a significant increase in births, seemingly at the expense of Morningside, particularly at the expense of the Wilkinson site.

Morningside's inability to stem the erosion in market share was based on one inescapable fact: the obstetrical program at Morningside lacked a comprehensive identity. Obstetrical care was being provided at two sites with very different philosophies, different methods of service delivery, and different types of facilities.

At Wilkinson, care was provided in a traditional manner in outdated physical facilities. Service delivery was based on a 1950s concept, the multitransfer system, which created psychological and physical risk by transferring patients at sensitive physiological times. The consequences were fragmented service and a lack of continuity of care. On the other hand, the hospital's special care nursery and the high-risk obstetrical program had been a center of excellence regionally and had enjoyed a national reputation for its innovative programs of care and its contributions to science. Physicians and hospitals throughout the state and surrounding states referred their patients to Wilkinson for high-risk care. The core tertiary services were offered within the special care nursery. In 1987, 261 admissions to the special care nursery were from the Bakerville metropolitan area; 481 were from the surrounding region. Physicians in the region referred patients to this perinatal program based both on its reputation as a center of excellence and on the professional relationships established with Morningside physicians. However, the special care nursery was housed in inadequate space; it was chronically overcrowded, at approximately 150 percent occupancy. The physical facility provided for approximately 40 square feet per bassinet (at average occupancy rates), whereas standards suggested an allocation of 120 square feet per bassinet. Electrical and mechanical systems were inadequate to support recent advances in neonatal care.

In contrast, the Birth Place at Lutheran Hospital was housed in more contemporary space and provided consumer-oriented care within a single birth room (that is, labor, delivery, and recovery in one room with separate postpartum facilities). However, the service was limited in the level of care it could offer. Its lack of tertiary services made it difficult for the program to grow and expand beyond the gains experienced in the previous ten years. A market survey from April indicated consumer preferences for obstetrical services.

The Search for an Identity

Dr. Boswell knew that Morningside needed to work on its identity problem. Before he could ask the hospital staff to concentrate on change, however, he needed to know more about the market. What kind of program would the community support? A market survey was conducted in April 1987 to elicit consumer perceptions of the ideal obstetrical program. The results of the survey indicated that consumers felt the ideal program should have several characteristics:

1. A broad range of services from low-intervention to high-risk birth
2. A residency program
3. Either the single room maternity care (SRMC) concept or the LDR concept
4. A variety of options for the birthing experience (such as rooming in, alternative birthing styles, extended visiting hours, and allowing the father to stay overnight in the mother's room)
5. A warm, homelike atmosphere created through interior design, furnishings, and lighting
6. Private baths

With this in mind, Dr. Boswell was ready to approach his staff and to ask them to work together and with him to come up with a solution to Morningside's problem.

On 2 June 1987, Tim Boswell had a breakfast meeting with Peter Flemming, M.D., Chief of Obstetrics at Wilkinson, and Nancy Fortune, M.D., Chief of Obstetrics at Lutheran. Dr. Flemming, a 57-year-old obstetrician, had practiced obstetrics-gynecology in Bakerville for 20 years. His practice was focusing more on gynecological surgery these days. Dr. Fortune, a 32-year-old obstetrician, had moved to Bakerville from northern California three years ago. The purpose of the meeting was to discuss the possible consolidation of perinatal services at Morningside.

Dr. Boswell began. "We don't have an identity yet at Morningside. Lutheran and Wilkinson each have their own identity, but since the merger Morningside has lost 5.5 percent of the market share to St. Catherine's. What should we do?"

Dr. Fortune responded first. "St. Catherine's Hospital obstetrics service is similar to Lutheran's, only it is newer and bigger. Wilkinson has a reputation with the childbearing population of the county for offering a high-tech and high-intervention obstetrics service. The cesarean rate is 16 percent as compared to ours at 8 percent. Lutheran offers nurse midwives. Our practice styles are very different. This is an educated community. Consumers know the difference and obviously want lower-tech, lower-intervention OB services. That's why they're going to St. Catherine's now. Since the merger, Lutheran has lost its consumer identity. People are confused."

Dr. Flemming piped in. "Hogwash. Wilkinson has an excellent regional reputation for high-risk services. Some of these mothers and babies wouldn't be alive today if it weren't for the advanced technology we offer."

"Another point you should remember," said Dr. Fortune, "is that St. Catherine's does not offer sterilization or pregnancy termination services."

"That's true," added Dr. Flemming. "Morningside does offer a complete OB-GYN service."

A week later, after deciding that he needed another perspective, Dr. Boswell invited Morningside's two head nurses to lunch. Martha Zimmerman, R.N., the head nurse from Wilkinson and a veteran of Vietnam, offered her thoughts.

"Dr. Boswell," she said, "I've delivered babies in the jungle, where there was no technology, and in luxurious hospitals of suburban Chicago, where there was only the best technology. I'd rather work with the best. This is the twentieth century. We've made so much progress and have saved so many more mothers and infants because of it!"

"Yes, but at what price?" asked Eileen Spiars, R.N., a certified nurse midwife. "Our society is pretty crazy. Why not put the emphasis on a family-centered philosophy, so infants can bond to their parents immediately after delivery? Let's strengthen the family unit. We don't have to sacrifice quality."

Dr. Boswell was not sure what to do. As the Birth Place experience at Lutheran had demonstrated, LDR with separate postpartum facilities was a program with high consumer appeal. It did not require major system changes or extensive cross-orientation of staff. The major drawback to this system, however, was that it did not achieve significant efficiencies in operating or staffing systems and it was no longer unique in the Bakerville area. If they implemented an LDR program, Morningside would only be playing catch-up with St. Catherine's and would not, in all probability, recapture the lost market share or acquire any new market share. Single room maternity care offered consumers the greatest number of options, promoted family-centered care and family participation in the birth event, achieved significant operating efficiencies, and was truly unique in the region. The major obstacles were the high start-up costs associated with renovation and cross-training of staff in all phases of obstetrical care.

The Retreat

Dr. Boswell planned a retreat to get a consensus on a plan of action for combining Lutheran's and Wilkinson's perinatal departments as Morningside's perinatal department. The retreat was scheduled for the first day of July, and the theme was "Form Follows Function."

The decision-making process was defined in a memo for the participants (see Appendix 11.2). Each participant would have equal status with all other participants in a consensus-oriented, nonvoting mode of meeting. The plan developed at the retreat would be submitted to the Morningside Hospital Board of Directors for approval and the ultimate decision on perinatal services would be made by the board. Dr. Boswell asked Fred Birmingham, a hospital planner, to assist the group.

As he sat pulling together the last details for the staff retreat, Dr. Boswell finally allowed himself to start imagining the future. He was thinking about how the board of directors would react to the final recommendations about the location, facility design, and type of obstetrical care to be provided by the new perinatal program at Morningside. It had been a year since the merger had taken place, and it was time to make some of the decisions necessary to extend the hospital consolidation effort beyond the perinatal department. The manner in which these decisions were made, as well as the final outcomes, would set the tone for all future decisions to be made on behalf of the newly merged hospital. Many stakeholders were interested in the outcome, and Dr. Boswell knew that he would need support from the board members and the individual contingencies that they represented.

Appendix 11.1: Summary Report on Maternity Services in the United States

A. Women are hospitalized more frequently in childbearing ages.

  1. Eighty or more women out of 100 are having their first child and will be back in someone's hospital in the near future.

  2. Cesarean deliveries increased by about 10 percent between 1970 and 1983, which means an increase in hospitalization days.

  3. Maternity is a growing market.

B. One in five "baby boom" women will probably end up childless. Infertility and increased procedures for childless couples will increase hospitalization.

C. Hospitalization was 17 percent higher for women than men in 1980, excluding deliveries. The surgery rate per 1,000 population was 81.3 percent for females and 55.1 percent for males.

D. On the average, women live about $7^{1}/_{2}$ years longer than men.

E. Women are influential in 90 percent of all health care decisions.

F. Fifty-eight percent of pregnant women choose a hospital first and a physician second for maternity care.

G. Thirty-eight percent of all families have their first encounter with a hospital through the maternity department.

H. The average pregnant woman visits three hospitals before choosing the one where she will deliver.

I. Women travel outside their community for health care. The market research conducted across the country indicates that women travel (sometimes for as long as one hour) for services they perceive to be special.

Appendix 11.2: Memo to Morningside Hospital Staff

DATE: June 20, 1987
TO: All Retreat Participants
FROM: Tim Boswell, M.D., Medical Director of Morningside
            Hospital
RE: Perinatal Retreat, July 1, 1987

The purposes for this retreat are as follows:

— To develop service design and then a facility to support the desired design

— To determine ancillary and support services needed to support the design

— To gain a consensus plan of action

— To bring all the practitioners together as one team

— To bring the current services together in an integrated system

— To eliminate the "we–they" barriers to enable all to practice in a collegial mode

— To develop an action plan and timetable, and to assign persons responsible for follow-up

One of the merger goals will be to integrate programs to achieve economies of scale. This goal does not predetermine the use of either the Lutheran or the Wilkinson facility, but it does mean that we will not operate two full-service general hospitals. We will continue to operate services at both facilities. Our challenge is to determine how best to allocate our services at each facility in order to meet the needs of our patients. Therefore, the retreat group's assumption that the hospital does not have sufficient capital finances to develop and maintain two complete perinatal sites and still meet its other financial requirements is correct. As we manage these changes, and others to come in the merger, we must continue our commitment to staff. We are committed to offering meaningful employment opportunities to all of our staff.

Yet to be determined are many other issues such as the location of all clinical services, including perinatal, and the way they will relate to one another. The retreat group is authorized to move forward on planning, and we hope to develop a detailed plan of action by the end of August. The planning process needs to include at least the following: market testing, space design and requirements, staffing requirements, a communications plan, and an implementation plan with stages for change.

The Morningside Hospital administration has made an 18-month commitment to Birth Place at the Lutheran Hospital. There will be no changes to the Birth Place program during that period of time. Morningside administration has budgeted a $2–3 million capital commitment and has directed that the perinatal plan will be completed within 18 months.

Governance at Lonetree and Prairie Group Practices

Blake E. Waterhouse, M.D.

This case took place in a stable midwestern community of about 350,000 people. The community experienced a 4 to 5 percent increase in population per year. The community boasted a strong health care system, with three private hospitals and one university hospital, a long history of strong medical group practices, and many solo practitioners and small specialty groups. Recently, there had been a marked increase in prepayment activity. Several HMOs had developed, predominantly revolving around each of the four hospitals in the community.

Two of the private hospitals were closely aligned with Lonetree Group Practice and HMO, one of two large group practices in town. The third private hospital had a more traditional medical staff mix and customary physician-hospital relationships with a separate medical staff group practice. Because of the increasing economic threat of the success of the two large group practices and their respective HMOs, the solo and small groups affiliated with the third private hospital joined together to start a third large group practice in the community and formed their own HMO, Prairie Group Practice and HMO. However, competitive pressures were prompting the leadership of the Lonetree and Prairie group practices and their HMOs to seriously consider a formal merger.

Lonetree Group Practice and HMO

Lonetree was a very successful and stable multispecialty medical clinic with a 70-year history. It had one central facility and two large satellites that shared a long history of unified decision making, shared governance, an income distribution formula, and medical records.

The physicians at Lonetree believed very strongly that the medical group should own and operate any HMO activity. However, they were discovering that a larger HMO patient base was needed to be actuarially sound. In addition, to make optimal use of the surgical subspecialists in the group, there needed to be an expanded base of primary care patients.

Organization of the Lonetree group

Ownership: The Lonetree group was physician owned. When each of the partners had become shareholders, they purchased an equal amount of stock at a consistent price. The buildings were held in a separate partnership and were also owned equally by each partner. Every physician was required to be both a partner in the building partnership and a stockholder in the corporation.

Governance: The shareholders elected a seven-physician board of directors. The board was elected by the entire group and did not represent specific departments or divisions.

Management: Management was the responsibility of a nonphysician administrative staff. There was a part-time medical director who attended all board meetings and reported to the board but was not a voting member of the board.

Size: There were approximately 60 physicians in this group practice.

Organization of Lonetree HMO

Ownership: The HMO was 100 percent owned by the medical group.

Governance: The medical group appointed five physicians and four public members-at-large to the nine-member board of directors.

Management: Management included a full-time administrative staff and a part-time medical director. The HMO was federally qualified and was not a for-profit entity.

Size: The enrollment was 17,000.

Prairie Group Practice and HMO

Prairie Group Practice and HMO was a relatively new face in the community. Its formation was accomplished after several months of difficult and rancorous discussion between the solo and small medical groups, all concerned about the economic strength of Lonetree and the town's other large group practice.

Organization of Prairie group

Ownership: All members of the new group purchased equal shares of common stock and were issued preferred stock in exchange for their office furnishings, and equipment.

Governance: The physicians elected a nine-member physician board of directors. The board was elected by the departments (or divisions) to represent their specific unit. The group was relatively unstable, with no history of shared governance, unified decision making, or common income formulas. There was no one central facility and there were 15 to 20 locations.

Management: Management included a nonphysician administrative team and a part-time medical director. The medical director was a full voting member of the board of directors.

Size: There were approximately 100 physicians in this newly formed group practice.

Organization of Prairie HMO

Ownership: The ownership of the HMO formed by this new medical group was shared equally by the medical group, the hospital, and an insurance company. Each owned one third of the HMO corporation.

Governance: The board of directors was composed of nine people, with three of the board members each appointed by one of the three owners.

Management: The management was almost exclusively undertaken by the insurance company. The HMO was for-profit and was not federally qualified.

Size: There were approximately 23,000 people enrolled in this new HMO, and almost all were previous patients of the physicians in the new medical group.

Merger Discussions

Preliminary merger discussions between Lonetree and Prairie were undertaken early in 1986. Both medical groups were interested in having larger HMO enrollments to allow for more accurate actuarial projections to minimize the financial risk of the medical groups. In addition, Lonetree was seeking an increased primary care base and more diverse geographical locations. Prairie wanted an enhanced surgical subspecialty mix and a more stable governance environment. The reimbursement climate at this time had the following characteristics:

1. Rapidly decreasing MAAC (maximum allowable acceptable charge) with increasing fees, resulting in widening disparities between physician bills and collected fees for those services. This discrepancy was most striking in the surgical subspecialties.

2. There was an increasing reliance on managed care reimbursement such as HMO, PPO, and government entitled programs. This accounted for approximately 50 to 60 percent of both groups' revenues.

3. Both medical groups had traditional fee-for-service income distribution formulas, with incentives for total billings (rather than collectable billings or rewards for efficiencies of managed care). Income statements and comparative statistics for both HMOs are presented in Appendixes 12.1 and 12.2. Each organization had a net worth of approximately $700,000.

After a great deal of analysis, both groups concluded that a merger would be mutually strategically beneficial but operationally very difficult. There were a number of issues that complicated the proposed merged entity, the combined clinics, and both HMOs. Among the issues that needed to be addressed were the following:

Merger of the practice groups

Ownership: There needed to be some recognition of the different levels of financial contribution that the previous entities had made to the ownership. The name of the merged entity was in question. All of the preexisting groups had name recognition and significant pride in their heritage. Some resolution had to be found for the differing levels of control and autonomy desired by the various entities.

Governance: The size of the board of directors, the selection process for the board, and the representative constituency of each board member had to be resolved.

Management: Physician versus nonphysician CEO decisions had to be made. The role of the medical director needed to be clarified. The role of the departments in both governance and operational issues had to be resolved. The selection of administrative staff was difficult since there were many duplications in positions in the preexisting medical groups.

The consolidation of operations would be difficult and had to include an income distribution formula, information systems, personnel policies, and pension plans, all of which were markedly different within the preexisting medical groups.

Merger of the HMOs

Ownership: Who should own the HMO? A few options were possible: physician ownership, partial ownership by the hospital, and ownership involvement by the insurance company.

Governance: The selection of the board of directors, the term of the board, and the mix of the board had to be determined.

Management: Decisions had to be made concerning whether the administration of the HMO would be internal or external to the medical group, whether the HMO would be for-profit or not-for-profit, and whether it would be federally qualified or not federally qualified. The selection and clarification of the role of the HMO medical director needed to be ironed out.

The following discussion took place one evening at a merger planning session:

LONETREE CEO: For continuity and stability, perhaps we should consider simply combining both preexisting boards for a period of two to three years.

PRAIRIE BOARD MEMBER: That would give Lonetree a disproportionate representation on the new board, based on the number of physicians in their group compared with the combined group. I believe we should hold new elections for all of the board positions and elect them by department.

LONETREE BOARD MEMBER: That would make no sense to me. Prairie has more physicians than Lonetree, and we might very well not have any of our previous Lonetree physicians elected to the new board of directors if we opt to elect all new board members.

PRAIRIE MEDICAL DIRECTOR: I believe it is important for the board to have departmental representation, which is the way the Prairie board was comprised. But since the Lonetree board was all elected from the membership at large, I don't see how we could combine the two previous boards even using the option of merging the old Prairie board with a portion of the Lonetree board.

PRAIRIE CEO: I believe it is critical for both previous groups to continue to feel represented, so perhaps we should consider the option of using all of the Prairie board members plus four of the Lonetree board members, which would be proportionate to the numbers of physicians in each organization, and do this with the understanding that after four to five years we would move to the option of electing all new members with departmental representation.

PRAIRIE BOARD MEMBER: I think four to five years is much too long. It gives Lonetree more representation than they should have. If we choose the proportional option, it should only be for one year of transition and then we should go to the option of electing all new board members by departmental representation.

The group decided that Dr. Alan Jackson, the Prairie medical director, would prepare a memorandum listing the strengths and weaknesses of all of the options and an implementation plan for the one he considered most feasible. Based on these considerations, the final decision would be made by the merger committee at the next meeting.

Appendix 12.1   Comparative Statistics, Lonetree and Prairie HMOs

	Lonetree HMO	Prairie HMO
Average number of members for period	10,205	21,610
Average number of physicians for period	66	235
Members per physician	154.62	91.96
Total ambulatory encounters	48,252	74,772
Ambulatory encounters per 1,000 members	4,728.27	3,460.06
Hospital days	3,043	9,815
Hospital days per 1,000 members	298.19	454.19
Inpatient admissions	698	1794
Inpatient admissions per 1,000 members	68.40	83.03
Average length of stay	4.36	5.47
Inpatient costs per admission	$1,847	$2,918
Average hospital cost per day of hospitalization	$423	$533
Revenue per member	$643	$688
Gain (loss) per member	$65.69	$8.65
Administrative cost per enrollee	$76	$58
Marketing costs as a percent of total premium	3.5%	5.2%
Marketing cost per enrollee	$21	$34
Marketing costs per affiliated physician	$3,331	$3,204
Marketing costs per clinic physician	$3,997	$3,126
Reinsurance cost per enrollee	$11	$14
Revenue per physician	$99,392	$63,288
Gain (loss) per physician	$10,157	$795
Profit margin	0.1022	0.0126
Total current enrollment	13,649	35,719

Appendix 12.2   Income Statements, Lonetree and Prairie HMOs

	Lonetree HMO	Prairie HMO
Revenue		
Premium	$6,177,099	$14,388,024
Fee-for-service	0	0
Copayments	32,410	0
Title XVIII (Medicare)	0	0
Title XIX (Medicare)	202,602	51,391
Interest	58,586	176,479
Coordination of benefits (COB) and subrogation	55,032	50,843
Reinsurance recoveries	34,169	205,838
Other revenue	0	0
Total revenue	$6,559,898	$14,872,575
Expenses—Medical and Hospital		
Physician services	$1,881,309	$ 6,870,318
Other professional services	632,875	553,029
Outside referrals	414,800	0
Emergency room, out of area	607,316	79,732
Occupancy, depreciation and amortization	0	0
Inpatient	1,289,377	5,235,722
Reinsurance expenses	114,914	302,704
Other medical	166,306	0
Incentive pool adjustment	0	149,248
Total (medical and hospital)	$5,106,897	$13,190,753
Administration		
Compensation	$ 0	$ 112,672
Interest expense	6,489	0
Occupancy, depreciation and amortization	25,358	2,630
Marketing	219,855	753,059
Other	530,907	388,795
Total (administration)	$ 782,609	$ 1,257,156
Total expenses	$5,889,506	$14,447,909
Income	$ 670,392	$ 424,666
Extraordinary item	0	0
Provision for taxes	0	237,772
Net income	$ 670,392	$ 186,894

Part V

Adaptation

Commentary

On Adaptation, Triceratops, and Strategic Choice

Robert B. Klint, M.D.

While walking south on Fifth Avenue in New York City, I was struck by the number of new street vendors. These are not the familiar magazine and newspaper sellers, warmed in permanent kiosks on nearly every corner. Rather, they are the sellers of watches, books, scarves, and after-shave lotions. Some seem ready for a quick exit, for their merchandise is displayed on cardboard boxes and blankets spread over the sidewalk. Others seem more permanent, approved by some municipal process that issues bright orange permits that dangle from their jackets. These entrepreneurs are selling calendars that are arranged in neat stacks upon portable tables with steel legs. The variety of calendars is impressive: dogs, cats, horses, birds of prey, and dinosaurs. There is more than one dinosaur calendar, so the purchaser has a choice of brontosaurus, allosaurus, tyrannosaurus rex, or triceratops. Next to the stack of reptilian calendars is one featuring a different endangered species for each month of the year. By the time I reached 42nd Street across from the public library, I must have passed two dozen stacks of dinosaur calendars.

Thirty-nine blocks to the south, near Battery Park, is the South Street Seaport, now restored to its early nineteenth-century splendor. In a corner shop, one can exchange $19.95 for an inflatable replica of a pterodactyl, a flying reptile whose 20-foot wingspan terrorized smaller creatures of the Mesozoic Era. The modern 36-inch variety can be hung in your child's playroom or your hospital's lobby as a reminder of the power of the evolutionary error.

Why all this fascination with the age of the reptiles? Those who labored through courses on paleontology were taught that these great and ponderous beasts somehow failed to evolve. They failed to change and adapt to a new environment. They had become too large and perhaps too specialized to survive in a changing world. Now, several years after taking Paleontology 101, we learn that the death of this order may have been quite sudden. The environment suddenly became cold, deprived of the chlorophyll-sustaining sunlight because of Earth's chance collision with a huge asteroid. There simply was not enough time for the brontosaurus to reduce its 60-ton mass and evolve into something else. It became outmoded and noncompetitive, and then disappeared. Dinosaurs and their flying reptilian cousins did not change.

A number of words can be used to describe such change: adjustment, conformity, versatility, compliance, adaptation, and evolution. Among these, the last two—adaptation and evolution—are frequently used to describe conditions in the health care industry. Yet, *evolution* seems unsuited for analogy to health care—too passive and reactive. *Adaptation*, on the other hand, better implies the deliberate action, thought, and planning that a craftsperson uses to adapt some tool for a new and different use. The cases in Part V are about change and adaptation in the health care environment.

The health care industry is reacting to profound changes in its world. In less than a decade it has felt the confusing, conflicting, and often overlapping policies first of regulation and then of competition. The proregulatory legislation of the 1970s produced the certificate of need, the professional standards review organization, and economic stabilization laws, each of which catalyzed later optimism for the prospective payment promises of the early 1980s. Dissatisfaction with the cost-containment outcomes and a leadership bias toward the benefits of competition produced changes designed to foster that competition. The U.S. Supreme Court approved advertising in health care. Growth of HMOs was stimulated with policy and funding. For-profit alternatives for delivering care were encouraged, and antitrust laws reached out to prove that health care players were no different from those in other industries. Yet the decade left millions uninsured, no clear policy on the effectiveness and availability of technology, many for-profit entrepreneurs among the unemployed, and growing public dissatisfaction with the system. Costs to health care purchasers increased 340 percent during the decade; competition reigned.

The competitive model has disappointed many due to its seeming inability to control costs, define the product, standardize treatment pro-

tocols, and ensure access to all who seek care. Some might place the
blame on the desks of the entrepreneurs whose much heralded entry
into the financial markets of Wall Street promised cost control through
competition and a fair market return on investment for all who believed.
Some would place the fault on the desks of health care leaders and in
the medicine bags of physicians, each of whom was unable or unwilling
to change.

Still others find fault with a legislature that was unwilling to address issues and a public convinced that technology could correct years
of making unwise, if not self-destructive, lifestyle decisions. In the
name of competition and building a better mousetrap, programs and
facilities have been duplicated, driving up the cost of care and threatening clinical outcomes. Nursing professionals left clinical nursing as both
the novice and the experienced were lured by other jobs and lifestyles.
Business leaders, recoiling from large increases in health benefit costs,
continue to push for discounts from providers while hospital providers
shift costs to finance care for the underinsured. Government shrinks
from its responsibility to provide either health policy or the funding
necessary to deliver on promises already made. Under failed social policy, the underinsured 13-year-old delivers her first baby and the fiscal
responsibility falls to institutions and medical staffs that are underfi-
nanced to provide the service. Some predict that one-third of all U.S.
hospitals will eventually close their doors.

Although some of these issues receive little public attention, the
expensive marvels of medical technology are widely acclaimed. The
evening news, lay journals, and other print media are replete with the
wonders of technology. Removal of gallstones without surgery, diagnosis without x-ray, coronary artery repair with balloons, and organ transplants of heroic proportions command public attention and support.
As demand for technology rises, a better-informed public is pursuing
wellness, prevention, dietary changes, and exercise, all of which are
changing the nature, frequency, and prevalence of major diseases.

Journals of the trade call for hospitals to renew their partnerships
with physicians, whose patient care decisions, referral patterns, and
practice habits significantly influence a hospital's financial well-being.
Slow to recognize its major customer, hospitals have developed bonding
strategies, established practice enhancement programs, and installed
computer networks in doctors' offices in order to attract and retain
physician customers. Many physicians cling to the nostalgia of fee-for-
service reimbursement while their hospital partners are paid at a fixed
rate. Economic policy seems to preclude collaborative and synergistic
procedures for delivering care.

This is the environment of the 1990s: a collage of high individual patient expectations, tremendous technological capabilities, inconsistent financial policy, labor shortages, growing pressure to reduce costs, growing need for defining, measuring, and improving quality, and a subliminal, gnawing feeling that somewhere the industry took the wrong evolutionary turn.

What responses are needed? Traditional contingency theory suggests that companies should alter their structures and behaviors to better meet an uncertain environment, which may require more creativity, more flexibility, and more innovation. In *The Art of War*, General Sun Tzu similarly coaches his generals, saying "when in difficult country, do not encamp. In country where high roads intersect, join hands with your allies. Do not linger in dangerously isolated places. In hemmed-in situations, you must resort to a stratagem. When there is dust rising in a high column, it is a sign of chariots advancing."[1] The victor must move quickly, often with small, well-focused, specialized forces who know their mission well. Knowledge of the terrain, flexibility, and a certain degree of guile help an army adapt to changing conditions.

Successful organizations, like maneuvering armies, become organic interactive organisms that sense, test, modify, and change. Organizational ecology demands that we make strategic and tactical choices. Some choices are less successful than others and should be dropped or modified. Choices that are successful during one time may not be successful during another. Organizations, like biological creatures, search for environmental niches where purpose, resources, and environment are most compatible.

What are the organizational strategies to be considered? R. E. Miles and C. C. Snow proposed a classification system for organizations based on their strategic choices. They created four categories: defender, analyzer, entrepreneur, and prospector. *Defenders* choose a narrow niche in a mature market. Competing principally on the basis of efficiency, they will move aggressively to maintain prominence in their chosen market segment. *Analyzers* also compete on the basis of efficiency but offer a broad range of products or services. Although ready to move into developing markets, these generalists rely on technical efficiency within an established and broad market domain. The *entrepreneurial* organization is the master at specialty and facileness, moving rapidly into new opportunities within a fairly narrow domain and utilizing swiftness to its advantage. The *prospector* is a generalist particularly skilled at finding and exploiting new broad markets. Each of these strategic types has its strengths and weaknesses; each can be more effective at different ages of market maturity. All can coexist successfully in an industry characterized by continuous and rapid technological evolution.[2]

Adaptation, then, is no passive evolutionary process of selection. Rather, it is an interactive contest requiring health care leaders to select a domain where resources are best employed, where survival and growth are most favored. Creativity, risk taking, and change management are among the tools to be used by the successful leader to proactively alter his or her organization. Significant changes have already begun. Health care organizations have created holding companies to facilitate change, started new businesses, and entered nontraditional markets.

Diversification strategies have spawned for-profit subsidiaries in home care, durable medical equipment, fitness centers, ambulatory care centers, women's centers, surgicenters, and more. Internal operations, policies, and procedures are changing. A language more commonly spoken on Wall Street is now heard in hospital board rooms in discussions of market share, business plans, profit centers, mergers, acquisitions, product line management, and equity-based joint venturing. Organizations look for their ecological and business niche. Some have attempted to become generalists by adding services and products to their holding company product lines. Others seek specialty niches through centers of excellence. For-profits and renegade entrepreneurs have seized opportunities in an expanded niche by entering the home care, durable medical equipment, and specialty hospital markets. These choices may be wise and necessary, but not all students of this transformation are comforted by it. "Where's the traditional mission?" they ask. "Where's the charity?" they wonder.

Goodwill, charity, care for the uninsured, humanitarianism, public health, and other goals of public good are still there, but they are well disguised by the need to compete, adapt, survive, and even flourish in a new and highly competitive marketplace.

Effective leaders cannot pause at the doorways to the external environment. In addition to guiding strategic choices for their own organizations, they should sketch a book of work that addresses fundamental questions about the industry. Quality standards need setting, overutilization needs pruning, the effectiveness of our technologies needs study and publication, a common agendum for physicians and hospitals needs setting, and more. A search for funding prevention and wellness as an alternative to the cost of repairing past damage must be completed. A voice that can speak to the capabilities of medicine and the constraints of business goals is needed to choose from among the trade-offs and choices that loom. Is the physician executive the next evolutionary genus?

The Part V Cases

Adaptation to such diverse and conflicting stimuli is difficult. Careful environmental scanning and a critical study of one organizational position and strategy is required. This portion of the book presents four case histories of institutions and the leaders who see a need to adapt and evolve into something better. In the first case, the medical director confronts changing demographics and a conflict of mission in an urban medical center. In the second case, the establishment of an IPA holds great promise for monitoring and delivering care, yet the effort is frustrated by the habits, beliefs, and financial interests of one group of stakeholders, the physicians. The third case describes a hospital and medical staff that wishes to create a new delivery model by sharing the risks and rewards of a joint venture but is hobbled by a lack of both trust and a process for goal setting. The last case asks the reader to develop a strategy for adaptation once a merger plan is frustrated by court action. Each case has in common the recognition that some new response to a segment of the environment is required for survival. Each case differs in its approach and tactics.

Overcrowding in the Midcity Medical Center emergency department

As urban population centers change in character, so do their corresponding urban health care institutions. Midcity was no different. Even though Midcity had only wanted to distinguish itself as a tertiary medical center, it found itself evolving from a general hospital to a subspecialized tertiary care center.

As primary care physicians moved their practices away from the downtown area, clinics became backlogged and poorly insured patients began relying upon the emergency department as their major source of primary care.

Case questions

1. What can Dr. Mitchell do to deal with the overcrowding problem in the emergency department?

2. Strategically, should Midcity exist primarily as a tertiary care hospital?

3. What role should Midcity play with regard to the medical care given to the downtown neighborhoods?

West IPA and Venture HMO (Part 2)

The relationship of West IPA to Venture HMO is akin to a dance in which each partner must step at the same time in beat to the music. If one partner cannot move in sync with the other, the dance is awkward and does not flow smoothly.

This case presents some clear-cut fiscal problems in a rapidly changing health care environment. The effects of these problems on physician practice is less clear. Dr. Evans has been given much data from Dr. Connor. He must sift through it to find out if it is the correct data to help him make a financial analysis. Is it enough information?

Case questions

1. What kind of data will be most useful to Dr. Evans?
2. Taking each of the problem categories of physicians ("upcoders," "churners," and "unbundlers"), recommend some specific ways to influence a change in their behavior.
3. What changes can be made concerning the hospital pool? The medical pool?

Joint venture?

Not only is Pineview Hospital trying to survive financially, but at the same time the administration is finding that it must play ball with the medical staff. Establishing joint ventures is one way to do both. The administration and medical staff struggle first with the definition of a joint venture and then with the choice of which joint ventures to pursue.

Case questions

1. What priorities do you, as the chief of the family practice department, recommend for the ten projects being considered as joint ventures? Why?
2. What information do you need to determine priorities?
3. Should the hospitals and physicians adopt a formal mechanism to deal with joint ventures, such as the traditional or the modular medical subject headings? Why?
4. If you had an opportunity to invest in the joint ventures for the preferred provider organization or the magnetic resonance imager, would you? Why?

5. What are the ethical considerations to be dealt with in joint ventures?

The Goodbody/LaGrange Merger:
What do you do when the judge says no?

After almost three years of planning for a merger between two hospitals in Fairview, U.S. District Court Judge Somewell put an axe to the entire plan. Massive amounts of time, energy, and financial resources had been spent on making the merger a reality. Relationships between the two hospitals had been unifying, identities merging, and trust was building. Overnight, the environment changed. All of a sudden the two hospitals became competitors again. The community was dismayed.

How is it possible for two massive entities to adapt when the legal system frustrates their long-range goals?

Case questions

1. Did the United States have any valid arguments for blocking the merger?
2. Did the Goodbody/LaGrange merger violate any antitrust laws?
3. Should the hospital appeal?

Notes

1. S. Tzu. *The Art of War*, edited by J. Clavel (New York: Dell Publishing, 1983).
2. R. E. Miles and C. C. Snow. *Organizational Strategy, Structure, and Process* (New York: McGraw Hill, 1978).

Overcrowding in the Midcity Medical Center Emergency Department

Richard L. Siegel, M.D.

Midcity Medical Center is a 525-bed, nonprofit hospital that was founded in 1910. Midcity is a large urban center, with a population of approximately 3 million. For the first 50 years of its existence, the medical center had the reputation of being the best acute care general hospital in the county. In the 1960s the board and the medical staff decided to concentrate on the creation and development of a number of specialty services (most notably, cardiology and cardiac surgery) with the intention of having these become tertiary referral services for the surrounding community hospitals. They felt this would distinguish Midcity Medical Center from the other acute care general hospitals in Midcity, thereby making it unique enough to maintain its reputation and, at the same time, provide the types of services that would ensure the hospital's financial viability.

They recruited a number of full-time, hospital-based specialists to become the chiefs of the clinical services and, at the same time, formed a teaching affiliation with State Medical School, also located in Midcity. This made the medical center one of the school's major sites for rotations of medical students, residents, and fellows in a variety of specialties and subspecialties, as well as an important center for clinical research in many of these areas.

By the early 1980s, the medical center had become the primary cardiac center in the state. The staff performed over 1,500 open-heart procedures per year and formed transfer agreements with almost all of the acute care general hospitals within a 25-mile radius. The full-time chief of surgery, Dr. D'Angelo, was also the chief of cardiac surgery. As such, he was one of the most respected and influential physicians on the medical staff. The focus of care gradually shifted and the medical center became a subspecialized, tertiary-level center, where the majority of patients being admitted were coming through referrals from primary care physicians in the surrounding communities to specialists either based at the hospital or on the hospital staff.

Mr. Madison, the medical center's chief executive officer since 1962, became aware that he was hearing more and more complaints from the general internists on the staff. One recurring complaint was that, when they would see a patient in their office who was complaining of symptoms compatible with a heart attack or unstable angina pectoris and would call the cardiac care unit (CCU) at the medical center to try to admit the patient, they would find that all the CCU beds were filled with the cardiologists' patients, many of whom were there for special or experimental procedures or drug protocols. The general internists would end up either sending the patient to the medical center's emergency department, where they would then have to wait in line for admission, or sending them to a CCU in one of the suburban hospitals where they had staff privileges and where bed availability was generally better due to less demand. Similar complaints were coming from the general surgeons, who were having increasing difficulty scheduling elective cases in the operating room because they were always competing for time with the cardiac surgeons.

Some of the more vocal of these physicians warned that, if they could not get the service they needed from the medical center, they would be forced to switch their affiliation and admit all their patients to the suburban hospitals. When a few of them actually did withdraw from the medical center's staff, the administration became increasingly sensitive to such threats. Although it was becoming clear to many observers that the medical center could not continue to function as both a general and a subspecialty hospital, the administration and the board were reluctant to give up the former and periodic concessions were made to the primary care physicians to try not to alienate them further.

Due to the medical center's physical location in the community and to the provisions of a number of its grants, it had developed a variety of outpatient clinics in adult medical and surgical areas, pediatrics, and women's health that were used primarily by area residents. Although these services were always adequate and provided an important source of patients for the medical school's training programs, they were never thought of as a priority. Because the majority of the hospital's revenues came from the subspecialty inpatient admissions, the emphasis had always been on developing these services and not the primary care ambulatory areas. As in many similar communities around the country, most of the primary care physicians preferred to have their offices in the more affluent suburbs rather than in the area immediately surrounding the medical center. Those whose offices were near the hospital were often reluctant to see patients who were poorly insured. As a result, many of the local residents were dependent on the medical center's clinics as their primary source of medical care. However, limited access to these clinics due to delays in scheduling appointments for acute or subacute problems led many people to use the emergency department for much of their primary care. Approximately 85 percent of the patients seen in the emergency department fell into the "semiurgent" or "nonurgent" categories, with the rest divided between "urgent" (10 percent) and "emergent" (5 percent).

The New Emergency Department Director

Dr. Robert Mitchell had completed a residency in emergency medicine and was a board-certified emergency physician. He had trained in an urban emergency medicine residency program, after which he had remained on the staff of the emergency department for approximately five years. During these years, he was heavily involved with the training of medical students and emergency medicine residents, and took an active role in the area's pre–hospital care (i.e., emergency medical service, or EMS) system. At about the time he was beginning to feel the need for greater administrative responsibility in his work, he was referred to Midcity Medical Center, and after several weeks of negotiations, he agreed to take the position as the medical director of their emergency department.

   Among Dr. Mitchell's first charges as the new director was to establish a group of full-time physicians to serve as the attending staff of the emergency department. He was able to accomplish this goal over the first two years of his term, while simultaneously phasing out most of the part-time positions that the department had previously depended on for physician staffing. There was now 24-hour-a-day coverage by full-time physicians (some of whom were trained in emergency medicine, others in other primary care specialties such as internal medicine and family practice). Double coverage was established during the eight hours each day when there were interns and medical students assigned to the department, so that one physician could be assigned to supervise these junior staff members.

In addition, Dr. Mitchell created a comprehensive set of policies and procedures for the department, established a nurse triage system to provide the initial evaluation of all patients who presented for care, redesigned the emergency department chart to allow for better documentation of medical, financial, and demographic data, and coordinated a rather extensive renovation effort to change the physical configuration of the department, in order to make the space more functional. He also designed and implemented a rather comprehensive quality assurance program for the emergency department, including a coordinated system for responding to patient complaints. During the first five years of his term as director, the emergency department successfully passed two site visits by the Joint Commission on Accreditation of Healthcare Organizations (JCAHO) and five annual inspections by the state health department, receiving no deficiencies from either regulatory body.

The Overcrowding Problem in Midcity's Emergency Department

The emergency department at Midcity sees patients with problems in all specialties (medicine, surgery, obstetrics-gynecology, pediatrics, and psychiatry). During the first year that Dr. Mitchell served as director of the department, they saw 37,500 patients. Over the next few years, the patient census in the department increased every year until, in the fifth year of Dr. Mitchell's term, the department was seeing approximately 45,000 patients per year. It was at about that time that Dr. Mitchell and the staff became aware that because inpatient beds were becoming less readily available, admitted patients were spending more and more time waiting in the emergency department for these beds. Dr. Mitchell began auditing and found that the problem was concentrated in the adult patients who were being admitted to the hospital's critical care units, which consisted of a 12-bed medical cardiac care unit, a 12-bed surgical cardiac care unit, a 48-bed cardiac telemetry/step-down unit, a 19-bed mixed medical/surgical intensive care unit, and a 10-bed respiratory care unit. When these are added to the numbers of beds in the pediatric and neonatal intensive care units, the medical center has the highest ratio of monitored to nonmonitored hospital beds in the state. Nevertheless, due to the hospital's tertiary referral status, these beds are frequently filled. The hospital generally follows a priority system for admission to these monitored beds. The highest priority goes to inpatients in medical/surgical beds who become acutely ill; next are patients admitted through the emergency department; next, patients being referred directly from physicians' offices for critical care admissions; and last, patients being transferred in from surrounding hospitals, for whom there are waiting lists for each of the above units. When a patient on a given unit is ready to be transferred to a general medical/surgical bed, thus freeing up their unit bed, if there are no patients in any of the first three categories waiting for it, a patient is called from that unit's waiting list and arrangements are made to transfer them to Midcity. Once such a call is made, the bed is considered to be occupied, even though it may take many hours for the patient to arrive.

When a patient has been evaluated in the emergency department and found to require admission to one of these units, the emergency department calls that unit directly. If such a bed is immediately available (which is rare), it is assigned to the emergency department patient and they are transported to it as soon as possible. If it is not available, the patient's name is placed on a waiting list for that unit, and the patient is called as soon as the next bed is vacated. Although a number of hospitals across the country—especially in the larger urban areas—have reported emergency department overcrowding with long delays in getting admitted patients to inpatient beds, most of these have been general, rather than subspecialty, hospitals in which most of the patients are waiting for general medical/surgical rather than critical care unit beds. Although Midcity shared some of the same problems that causes this to occur in other hospitals (e.g., a shortage of inpatient nurses, resulting in beds sometimes having to be closed), its status as a tertiary center made its overcrowding problem somewhat unique and the result of a different set of causes.

In his investigation into the problem, Dr. Mitchell learned several interesting facts. Patients were almost never being transferred off the critical care units to unmonitored medical/surgical beds until their unit bed was needed for another patient. As a result, these unit beds were almost always occupied. The reasons for this were twofold: First, the staff physicians felt that, because of the higher nurse-to-patient ratio on the units compared to the general medical/surgical floors, their patients received better care on the critical care units, regardless of whether or not the patient's problem justified keeping them there. Second, a physician could charge a higher visit fee for a patient on a critical care unit than for the same patient in a general medical/surgical bed. Therefore, there was no real incentive for the physicians to voluntarily transfer their patients off these units, and most of them waited until they were forced to do so.

To accomplish this, the nurses on the unit would first contact the resident or fellow assigned to the unit. The resident or fellow, in turn, would begin to contact the attending physicians of the patients who were acknowledged to be the least acute and, therefore, the best candidates for transfer off to a nonmonitored floor, as it was necessary to get the physician's consent prior to such a transfer. Depending on how quickly these physicians would respond and how many would have to be called before one agreed to allow their patient to be transferred, this process could go quickly or could be very time-consuming.

Once the process was started, the unit would then have to contact the admitting office to find out if a medical/surgical bed were available. Not uncommonly, this would be an additional source of delay. Either there truly were no unmonitored beds available (i.e., the hospital was at 100 percent occupancy) or there were patients whose physicians had given consent for them to be discharged but were delayed in leaving their rooms (e.g., because they had no means of transportation home). To Dr. Mitchell's knowledge, the hospital's mandatory discharge time of 10:00 A.M. had never been enforced. The policy was treated casually since there was already a perceived reluctance on the part of patients to come to Midcity, and the administration did not want to do anything that might further alienate these patients.

After a room was found and the patient transferred, the unit bed would have to be prepared by the housekeeping staff. The staffing for housekeeping was variable, with only a skeleton crew on the night shift although there were almost always patients admitted at night through the emergency department. Dr. Mitchell also learned that there was no system in place to inform the housekeepers when a room needed cleaning, so nursing staff on the unit had to call and request them to come. There was no record of such calls and, therefore, no way of determining whether the requests were handled expeditiously or not. Dr. Mitchell heard frequently from the emergency department nursing staff that they often would call housekeeping themselves when patients were waiting for these rooms, only to learn that the unit's nursing staff had not informed them that a bed was waiting to be cleaned.

Dr. Mitchell did an audit of the previous three months' admissions to the critical care units, dividing them into those admitted before 5:00 P.M. and those admitted after 5:00 P.M. He learned that there was never a night during this period when fewer than three patients were admitted through the emergency department to one or more of these units, and that many of these admitted patients waited in the emergency department all night before a bed became available the next day.

With the assistance of the hospital's quality assurance department, Dr. Mitchell was able to extract information from the hospital computer system to look at the utilization of beds on the critical care units, especially the telemetry/step-down unit. He concentrated on this unit because his monthly audits showed that these were the beds for which the emergency department consistently waited the longest, as patients were frequently admitted there directly from the emergency department for cardiac problems that were clinically stable. He found out that 36 percent of all the patients who spent time on this unit were discharged directly to home, rather than first going to a nonmonitored medical/surgical bed. His concern was that, for some percentage of these patients, a discharge order was written the evening or night before the day they were going home. The implication was that, if necessary, these patients could have been transferred off the unit to a regular floor bed for the last night, which would have opened up their telemetry unit bed for another emergency department patient who was waiting for it.

The Two-Hour Bypass

Midcity Medical Center is a receiving hospital for a number of local ambulance companies, including a municipal service in Midcity and several private and volunteer companies, both in Midcity and in several surrounding communities. Some of these have only basic life-support ambulances, while others include advanced life-support vehicles. The medical center administration made the decision a number of years ago that it did not want to have its own ambulance service, partly because it would be more of an expense than a source of additional revenue, and partly because there was more interest in receiving specialty care patients than the patients with more general medical and surgical problems, most often brought in by ambulances that respond to the public.

A few of the ambulance companies have their own dispatchers, but most of them are linked by Midcity's 9-1-1 system through a central dispatch center, which provides a coordinated system of response to calls for ambulances within the city limits. This system includes a method for diverting ambulances away from emergency departments or hospitals whose resources are temporarily filled to capacity. Each institution in the system reports its status on a regular basis to the EMS dispatch center.

At Midcity Medical Center, there are several categories of diversion. When the emergency department is temporarily overcrowded, they can request a two-hour bypass, either limited to critical care patients or to include all patients who might be brought by ambulance. When the hospital's critical care units are unable to accept additional patients, an eight-hour critical care diversion can be implemented to prevent patients in this category from being brought in. Similarly, when there are no available adult beds in the entire hospital, an eight-hour full hospital diversion can be initiated.

Although this system had only been used by Midcity EMS for two years, statistics showed that the medical center had instituted a two-hour bypass (due to emergency department overcrowding) more frequently than had any of the other hospitals in the system. Periodically, Dr. Mitchell received a note from Mr. Madison, Midcity's CEO, asking him whether anything could be done about this, usually after Mr. Madison had received a complaint from a physician on the medical staff about a patient who had been taken by ambulance to another hospital while the emergency department was on bypass.

Thinking that it might strengthen his stance on solving the overcrowding problem, Dr. Mitchell did an analysis of the financial impact of the emergency department's use of ambulance diversion. Using the frequency with which various categories of diversion or bypass had been instituted over the past six months, and combining this with both the average number of critical care admissions (via ambulance) in a 24-hour period and the DRG rates of reimbursement for these types of admissions, Dr. Mitchell calculated that the hospital was losing approximately $750,000 in revenue annually as a result of the potential admissions lost by diverting ambulances. Dr. Mitchell did not share this information with anyone.

The Problem-Solving Discussion

In considering how best to approach the situation, Dr. Mitchell invited the key players to a meeting one morning and asked each to summarize their concerns. The following discussion took place.

Mr. Madison (CEO): I understand Dr. Mitchell's position. As the director of the emergency department, he is concerned that patient care and staff morale may be suffering as a result of overcrowding. In theory, I know it makes sense not to keep bringing patients to the emergency department when there is nowhere to put them and not enough staff to take care of them adequately. However, you have to understand my position as well. I have to think about the fact that, by pushing the doctors harder to discharge their patients from the critical care units or creating rules that say they must do this under certain conditions, I risk having them tell me it's too difficult to work here and either start sending their patients elsewhere or possibly even withdrawing from the staff altogether. The same thing applies to continuing the present ambulance diversion system, where patients of doctors on the staff here end up being taken to other hospitals because we're closed to ambulances. When these doctors tell me that they don't have this problem at the other hospitals they admit to, what am I supposed to tell them? In addition, I suspect that, by diverting ambulances and sending away potential admissions, we may even be losing revenue, although I haven't had the time to sit down and analyze this to see if it's true.

MR. WHITLIN (Associate Director): I've heard both sides of the argument and I'm convinced that we have to push for better controls in our own internal systems. Things like mandatory discharge times and standard, enforceable criteria for transferring patients out of critical care units have worked in other hospitals; I see no reason why they wouldn't work here. It would involve a transition period during which everyone would have to get used to some new ways of doing things. It may ruffle a few feathers but I think that, if people see the guidelines being applied equally to everyone across the board, and if it results in a more smoothly running operation—which I think will be the case—I believe the vast majority of people, including the physicians, will accept it. I think too much is made of the threats we hear from a vocal minority of the doctors. I think most of them are too tied into our system to want to start trying to build a whole new referral base in another hospital. You know, those other hospitals have plenty of other doctors who may not welcome them with open arms.

DR. D'ANGELO (Chief of Surgery and Cardiac Surgery): Since I came to this hospital in 1965, I've always considered the emergency department to be an important component. Although I have very little contact with it in my day-to-day practice, it's important for me to feel that, on the occasions when my patients do get acutely ill, I can tell them to come to the emergency department here and feel comfortable that they will receive good care. In addition, with more than 40,000 visits per year, a lot of people's first impressions of the medical center are formed in the emergency department. These impressions last, and they can make it either easier or more difficult for us to deal with these patients afterward. Dr. Mitchell has done a damned good job of getting the department into the kind of shape where it is capable of serving this function. Now we have to support him to make sure that we (the medical staff) are not contributing to problems that are making it impossible for the department to do its job well. After all, it's to our benefit for it to work. It disturbs me when I see physicians acting in a self-serving manner by subverting the system to get something they need. Granted, each of us is supposed to be an advocate for our own patients, but when doing this means disrupting the running of the rest of the hospital, it can't be tolerated. I've told Dr. Mitchell that I want to help him try to get the medical staff to cooperate in solving his problems, and I mean it.

DR. JOHNSON (President of the Medical Staff): It's hard enough to practice medicine today with all the new rules and regulations coming from every direction and someone always telling you what you can and can't do. The hospital has to try to make it as easy as it can for the physicians to function within this framework. When we get harassed in the middle of our office hours about transferring patients off the telemetry units or discharging patients to go home, when we know we're going to be coming down in a few hours to make our rounds and will be able to take care of these things then, we end up resenting it. I've talked with Dr. Mitchell about the overcrowding problem and I get copies of most of the memos he writes to the administration and the other clinical chiefs about it. I can sympathize to a certain extent, but I don't feel that he really understands what we are up against as private practitioners who are mostly in office-based practices. I don't know how serious most of the threats are that I hear about doctors leaving the staff. However, I do think it's a sign of the frustration a lot of us feel at what we have to go through to practice here.

DR. WAGNER (Chief of Cardiology): I am faced with a rather difficult situation that I don't know if Dr. Mitchell fully appreciates. Where I trained and practiced prior to coming here, 60 to 70 percent of the cardiologists in the division were hospital based, with some formal affiliation to the hospital, including arrangements for sharing income and expenses. This made it much easier for the chief of cardiology there to have more authority over what these physicians could or couldn't do. Here, the division is comprised of about 10 percent hospital-based cardiologists, with the other 90 percent being private practitioners in office-based practices, over whom I have much less control. The expectations of the majority are high when it comes to services they want from the hospital, and most of them have become very adept at gaming the system, and that includes waiting to discharge a patient from a telemetry bed until they have another one of *their* patients to admit to that bed. Things like this are clearly unfair and are the type of thing that undoubtedly contributes to the problems Dr. Mitchell is facing in the emergency department. However, they are very difficult for me to control. If I become too heavy-handed and start disciplining people for these infractions of the rules, they always have the option of taking their patients to other hospitals. Since they already get most of their referrals from primary physicians in the surrounding communities, this would not be as difficult for them to do as it would for some of the primary care physicians. Although the medical center's tertiary capacity clearly offers certain advantages to these physicians, I'm afraid that this could easily be counterbalanced by subjecting them to too many hassles.

MS. GREEN (Nurse Administrator, Emergency Department): I've worked with Dr. Mitchell now for seven years and have come to respect him both as a physician and as a department head. However, remember that I've been in this hospital for over 25 years and in this department for 15 years, so I think I have a pretty good perspective on the situation. I can honestly say that I have never seen the morale among the emergency department nurses as low as it is now. Tempers are short, and the nurses are less able to deal as well with the day-to-day pressure than they used to be. In my opinion, this is clearly due to our overcrowding problem. The staff just feels overwhelmed too often. They're expected to deliver a level of care that they know we are not set up for. They have told me that they often feel like they are just plugging holes in a dike, waiting for it to spring a leak somewhere else. They're concerned about their licenses being in jeopardy because they know that they're being asked to do too much and that this will lead to forgetting something they were supposed to do or making some other type of mistake that may result in harm to a patient. In addition to seven vacancies, out of a total of 26 staff nurse positions, I have had a position open for an assistant head nurse for three months. That has never happened to me before. There was always a staff nurse who would be interested in the position. Now, none of them want the additional responsibility. To me, that's a sign of a problem that I'm afraid will get worse if nothing is done about the overcrowding situation.

Dr. Mitchell thanked everyone for sharing their concerns and proceeded to formulate a strategic plan for the emergency department.

Case 14

West IPA and Venture HMO (Part 2)

Anthony R. Kovner

Venture HMO, an investor-owned corporation, operates in a mid-Atlantic state through physician organizations known as individual practice associations (IPAs). Each IPA is a corporation that contracts with Venture HMO on behalf of its physician members to provide the services of private practice physicians. These IPAs enable individual physicians to care for their patients in the traditional manner—providing services in their own offices and being compensated on a fee-for-service basis.

Venture HMO's membership grew from 4,000 in 1979 to 168,000 in 1989. Eight IPAs and over 2,000 physicians participate in the system (see Table 14.1). Revenues for 1988 were $60 million and net revenue was $1.2 million or $0.40 per share. West IPA has 35,000 members and 350 affiliated physicians. It has a seven-member governing board elected by its affiliated physicians and meets once a month.

Paul Strauss, M.D., is a family practitioner and has been the president of West IPA since 1983. He devotes three hours per week to administrative work for which he is paid by the IPA. In 1987, Bill Evans, M.D., an internist, replaced Cynthia Anderson, M.D., who had been ineffective as the medical director of West IPA. Dr. Evans is paid 30 percent of a full-time-equivalent salary by the IPA to be the medical director. (For a job description of the West IPA Medical Director, see Appendix 14.1.) He spends one and one-half days per week on activities related to monitoring the cost and quality of care provided by West IPA physi-

This case is a sequel to A. R. Kovner, "West IPA and Venture HMO," in *Health Services Management: A Book of Cases* 3d ed., ed. A. R. Kovner and D. Neuhauser (Ann Arbor, MI: Health Administration Press, 1989), 136–40.

Table 14.1   Venture HMO: IPAs and Membership, 1988

IPA Physician	# of Members
1. Clark	15,000
2. David	30,000
3. Osler	27,000
4. Rouge	18,000
5. West	35,000
6. Lyons	22,000
7. Black	16,000
8. Green	5,000
Total	168,000

cians. In addition, Venture HMO pays West IPA approximately $25,000 per year for administrative expenses.

Hospital Pool

During 1988, West IPA spent $9 million for hospital care, well over the $8.2 million budgeted for the period. This resulted in a shortfall to Venture HMO of $800,000 for hospital care. Between 15 and 30 percent of total physician fees to West IPA physicians are withheld to pay for possible overages in hospital expenditures. The withholding varies depending upon which of the six hospitals in the area are used by West IPA physicians. Fifteen percent is withheld from physicians using the two hospitals that offer a discount to Venture HMO. Thirty percent is withheld from physicians when they admit patients to the other four hospitals. Despite the lower withholding for preferred hospitals, Dr. Strauss estimates that one-third of West physicians still admit their patients primarily to the hospitals that do not offer the discount to Venture HMO.

Medical Pools

West IPA physicians were over budget on both the physician pool and the miscellaneous pool. For 1988, this amounted to $900,000 for the physician pool and $400,000 for the miscellaneous pool. Thus, of the $1.4 million budgeted for withholding, to be paid back to physicians if these pools were on target, only $100,000 was available to be distributed for 1988 (see Table 14.2).

Sam Silus, M.D., a professional practice consultant to Paul Connor, M.D., the medical director for Venture HMO, stated that the principal

Table 14.2   West IPA: Risk Pools, 1988

	Cost
Medical Pool	
Budgeted	$8.0 million
Cost	8.9 million
Balance	($900,000) or $2.14 per member per month
Miscellaneous Pool	
Budgeted	$1.8 million
Cost	2.2 million
Balance	($400,000) or $0.95 per member per month
Withholding	
Withholding	$1.4 million
Pool overages	1.3 million
Withholding available	$100,000

causes of the medical pool shortfall in 1988 were the utilization practices of particular physicians. He classifies these physicians and their practices into three types: "up-coders" are physicians who charge for services that are more intensive than appropriate; "churners" are physicians who bring patients back and have a high referral rate to specialists; and "unbundlers" are physicians who break out services into separate subservices and charge for each subservice an amount much greater than a comprehensive service fee for the same care. In addition, the miscellaneous pool shortfall is related to excessive emergency department utilization, referrals to hospital outpatient laboratory, x-ray, and physiotherapy departments that do not offer discounts to Venture HMO.

There is a substantial difference in the pool costs between the physicians in West IPA and all of the physicians in Venture IPA groups. There is also a great variation in costs among specific West IPA physicians as shown in Table 14.3.

Dr. Evans has tried to understand why the practice of four West IPA physicians varies so greatly from that of the other West and Venture physicians (see Tables 14.4–14.7). He requested claim report summaries from Dr. Connor on these four physicians and received several reports from which Tables 14.4–14.7 are abstracted. Table 14.4 compares physician medical costs for seven selected services; Table 14.5 compares patient intensity, cost, and visits for selected physicians; and Tables 14.6 and 14.7 compare types and intensity of office visits, and costs and numbers of both visits and office procedures among selected physicians.

Table 14.3   Venture HMO and West IPA: Pool Costs, 1988

	Cost per Member per Month		
	Hospital	Physician	Miscellaneous
Venture (all physicians)	$23.34	$23.46	$ 4.76
West (GPs and FPs)	26.41	25.85	5.59
West MDs (selected GPs and FPs)			
Kahn	65.32	35.36	11.47
Demo	86.57	39.98	9.48
Oprah	52.86	52.38	20.47
Umble	68.16	39.49	10.23

Note: GP = General practitioners; FP = Family practitioners.

Table 14.4   Physician Costs for Selected Services
(per member per month)

	Venture HMO (all)	West IPA (all)	Selected Physicians			
			Kahn	Demo	Oprah	Umble
Periodic physical	$ 0.57	$ 0.86	$ 0.37	$ 0.46	$ 0.35	$ 1.10
Physician office visit	7.71	8.17	7.68	12.20	21.77	9.00
Physician hospital visit at SNF	1.63	1.95	6.06	8.71	7.40	3.13
Surgery	5.24	5.86	8.84	6.69	7.55	12.15
Ophthalmological exam	0.31	0.48	0.28	0.29	0.47	0.61
X-ray (part of office visit)	1.41	1.67	2.82	1.44	4.07	1.47
OPD lab/x-ray	2.01	2.54	7.06	4.22	9.67	4.57
Total	$18.88	$21.53	$33.11	$34.01	$51.28	$32.03

Note: SNF = Skilled nursing facility; OPD = Outpatient department.

Dr. Evans has reported to the IPA board and to Dr. Connor the following information based on his communication and interaction with the physicians:

> The *up-coders* say they need to spend enough time with their patients. They say they have sicker patients and that more of the visits of these patients are not routine. They practice quality medicine. They don't refer as many patients as other physicians do, and they spend more time with patients convincing them that they don't need specialist care.

Table 14.5 Intensity, Cost, and Number of Visits per Member (comparing standard and selected physician performance)

	Office Visit Intensity		Cost per Encounter	Cost per Referral Encounter	Encounters per Member per Year	Referrals per Member per Year
	New Patients	Established Patients				
(Standard)	14.66	5.64	$35.31	—	2.50	—
Kahn	9.01	5.21	53.16	$149.30	2.21	1.03
Demo	14.19	5.96	54.15	97.01	1.62	1.62
Oprah	17.04	6.11	39.96	123.71	4.33	3.57
Umble	17.05	7.10	43.90	127.71	1.41	2.17

Table 14.6 Profile of Office Visits: Type and Intensity (1/1/88 through 12/31/88)

Physi-cian	Panel Size	Office Visit Code										
		0	10	15	20	30	40	50	60	70	80	88
Kahn	352	0	30	0	5	0	0	688	9	0	0	50
Demo	249	0	15	0	30	2	0	262	390	2	1	25
Oprah	87	0	1	0	21	0	0	105	211	23	8	15
Umble	126	0	0	0	17	0	0	11	63	37	0	6

Note: The code structure is as follows:
0–20 = New patients (minimal, limited, intermediate, and comprehensive visits);
30–80 = Established patients (minimal, brief, limited, intermediate, extended, and comprehensive visits);
88 = Periodic physical.

Table 14.7 Profile of Office Visits: Cost and Number (1/1/88 through 12/31/88)

Physician	Panel Size	Average Intensity	Average Cost per Visit	Visits per Member per Year	Procedures per Code		
					850	870	930
Kahn	352	5.41	$ 5.34	2.08	30	35	60
Demo	249	6.54	79.40	2.83	85	35	30
Oprah	87	7.04	130.86	4.26	74	40	45
Umble	126	8.69	43.20	1.06	8	5	2

Note: The procedure code structure is as follows: 850 = Blood studies; 870 = Throat cultures; 930 = EKGs.

The *churners* say they must see the patient more to ensure that they are being monitored properly. They say they are afraid of malpractice suits. They practice high-quality care. They choose to have their offices close to nearby hospitals, so patients can be referred there for diagnostic studies, rather than near other IPA physicians or contracted facilities. Churners refer more patients to specialists because they say they are not experts in all aspects of medicine.

The *unbundlers* say they do not provide ordinary care. They say they spend more time with each patient than other doctors do. They perform all tests and procedures necessary and do not understand why they cannot provide the services that are essential to making diagnostic decisions. They are worried about malpractice suits and wish to provide high-quality care.

Dr. Evans has been told by the board of West IPA that there are cost overruns, that he has got to do something to reduce costs, and that he can ask Venture HMO for more data. Dr. Evans believes he is already getting too much data and not in the format that is most useful. Dr. Connor agrees that the format could be more streamlined but says changes have already been made in this direction. He adds that Dr. Evans and the IPA board have the data they need and that they are not doing enough to control medical utilization and cost.

Appendix 14.1: West Individual Practice Association Medical Director Position Specifications

Reports to: President, IPA
              Board of Directors, IPA

Responsibilities:

The responsibilities of Medical Director include but are not limited to the following:

1. Serves as a liaison between the IPA and HMO, and provides input for joint IPA/HMO committee functions.
2. Serves as chair of the IPA Quality Assurance/Peer Review Committee, and develops criteria and implements physician peer review and education programs.
3. Serves as a member of the HMO Standards Committee.
4. Devotes at least four (4) hours per week at the HMO office or by telephone, and as otherwise needed, to the following:

a. Reviews documents regarding medical necessity for hospital admissions on a prospective and concurrent basis, interacting with the admitting IPA physician as necessary.

b. Reviews hospital charts retrospectively and concurrently to determine the medical necessity of the admission.

c. Sends medical determination letters to physicians and other appropriate parties.

d. Screens requests for patient referrals (in and out of area).

The number of hours set forth above shall be reviewed periodically but at least annually, and shall be adjusted from time to time to reflect the needs of the IPA. Any such adjustment shall be accompanied by an appropriate adjustment to salary.

5. Reviews hospital, outpatient, and office claims for physician service to evaluate the utilization of services provided, the determination of reimbursement, and medical necessity.

6. In conjunction with the HMO Vice President, Professional Affairs, coordinates the development of medical policies and procedures.

7. Reviews and initiates action related to patient and physician grievances.

8. Recommends IPA reimbursement alternatives and schedules to the IPA.

9. Assists in recruiting physicians, and reviews and assists in making recommendations regarding the credentialing of physicians for membership in the IPA.

10. With the HMO Vice President, Professional Affairs, develops medical audit and medical care evaluation studies in furthering the development of the IPA.

11. Assists in the development and use of management information systems and data bases from such systems.

12. Develops written reporting document(s) for the board of IPA, on a regular basis, detailing Medical Director activities.

Qualifications:

1. License to conduct the practice of medicine in this state.

2. Sensitivity and background to analyze and respond to specialized HMO development issues.

3. The ideal Medical Director should not be an IPA board member but should be a salaried employee of the IPA and a primary care physician possessing a wide knowledge of medical and surgical practices. He or she should be comfortable in the medical/administrative/business world, possess a facility with numbers, be a good written and oral communicator, relate well to people, and be willing to make difficult decisions regarding the appropriateness of actions taken by peers.

Joint Venture?

Jerry Rose, Karl Merkle, M.D., and Fred J. Barten

Pineview Hospital is a 650-bed facility situated in the Midwest city of Heartford, the headquarters of a major automotive company and a large automobile manufacturing plant. The hospital is the second largest employer after the auto company in a city with a population of 96,000. It is also the largest supplier of health care services to the citizens of Heartford and the surrounding communities, with a service area of 800,000 people. The hospital has shown a surplus each year over the past five years, but net revenue is declining and competitive pressures make the future uncertain. Funds for equipment and construction are difficult to identify.

The auto company is a major employer of the patients in this service area. In the past they were generous in the purchase of health care packages for their employees. When the health care benefit package became too expensive, management started looking for alternatives to the more expensive Blue Cross/Blue Shield coverage. By late 1985, management's decision to cover their employees' health care needs was largely dependent on the availability of alternative delivery systems.

Originally prepared for the Institute in Administrative Medicine, University of Wisconsin–Madison, June 1987. Collaborators were Jerry Fitzgerald, Jerry Hoskins, and Carl Galiardi, M.D.

A PPO Business Proposal

In early 1986, the management of Pineview Hospital, sensitive to changes in the auto company and sensing an opportunity, enlisted two other suburban hospitals of similar size (600 and 1,000 beds) to join in a common effort to develop a preferred provider organization (PPO) and market health care to the large employers in their respective service areas. The service areas of the three institutions were complementary, covering a large metropolitan area.

The medical staffs of the three hospitals were made up of individual private practitioners. The majority of these practitioners, who were not favorably disposed toward alternative delivery systems, had to be brought into the fold to make the new plan marketable. The groundwork was laid by establishing a PPO committee at Pineview Hospital to encourage open discussion and dissemination of information about the joint effort. As a result of the committee's work, medical staff members and leadership became increasingly sensitized to the changes in the health care delivery system. Long discussions about the advantages and disadvantages of PPOs and HMOs ensued. The PPO was found acceptable as an alternative or addition to the private practice mode.

After administrative staff from the three hospitals had negotiated an agreement and established a business plan, representative members of the medical staffs of the three hospitals were invited to a presentation. The business plan was found lacking. It appeared that the physicians were to be used strictly as a tool to accomplish the hospitals' goals (i.e., to maintain or increase occupancy rates). Nothing in the plan made it attractive to the physician population.

A PPO Joint Venture Proposal

Physicians essentially walked out of the discussions of the plan. They hired their own legal counsel for the purpose of establishing a joint PPO venture with the institutions. It was apparent to the physicians that many of their patients would shift from their present insurance coverage to the PPO, so initially the physician patient load would be only minimally affected. It was apparent to the institutions that without the physicians' cooperation the plan was doomed to failure. It was the commonality of interest that started to drive this venture. Both the physicians and the institutions were seeking an opportunity for financial involvement in the corporation and an equal representation in the governance of that company.

To that end, six guidelines for the joint venture were proposed by the officers of the Pineview medical staff to develop the joint venture:

1. Hospital administration will be educated to the realities of a joint venture. (Without adequate numbers of physicians participating in the PPO, there would be insufficient numbers of patients.)

2. This educational process will be accomplished through the use of legal counsel for negotiations.

3. Stock *A* will be created for the hospitals and stock *B* for the physicians. The price of each is $15.75 per share, and they are to be sold in 100-share blocks.

4. Stock *B* will be marketed and sold to the physicians of the three institutions. A minimum of 50 participating physicians in each hospital will be required for the hospital to be represented on the board of the corporation.

5. Stock ownership is not necessary for physician participation in the PPO.

6. Governance of the corporation (Unified Health Services) will be shared equally between the hospital and the physician stock owners.

An MRI Proposal

Meanwhile, a proposal for a magnetic resonance imaging center was beginning to take shape. The MRI joint venture discussions were initiated by a staff neurologist in September of 1985. A total of 170 general partner units were offered at $10,000 per unit. In addition, the general partners planned to publicly offer and sell 100 limited partnerships each. The total capital anticipated was $2.7 million.

The MRI Management Committee would include nine individuals to hold most of the power of general partners: four from the hospital, two from the radiologists likely to become partners, two from remaining partners, and a ninth member appointed by the majority vote of the eight. Members would have as many votes as the general partners appointing them.

Joint Venture Proposals

By mid-1986, the senior administration at Pineview had "conversations" or "preliminary planning discussions" in process for nearly 40 joint venture projects, including these:

1. A physician office building
2. A freestanding laboratory
3. A malpractice/risk management program
4. A fourth ambulatory care center
5. A sports medicine program
6. A durable medical equipment manufacturer
7. A geriatrics center
8. A loan program to relocate new physicians in one of the three existing ambulatory care centers

Proposals for some of the programs, such as sports medicine, were initiated by physicians. Other projects, such as the office building and the loan program, were initiated by the hospital. Still others, like the malpractice/risk management project proposal, were initiated jointly by physicians and the hospital.

The number, scope, and timing of the proposals had become a problem. Should the proposals be reviewed on an ad hoc basis? Should there be a review process and protocol similar to review of research proposals? Who should be involved—the present medical staff officers and organization or an outside corporate group? The following conversation took place one noon in the hospital dining room:

CHIEF OPERATING OFFICER: What are we going to do about all of these projects being proposed as joint ventures? They are coming in from all over the organization and it's difficult to know what we are dealing with.

CHIEF FINANCIAL OFFICER: The MRI proposal sounds good to me. We are going to have to buy one ultimately anyway, and I'd be pleased to share some of the return, if there is any, in exchange for the capital from the physicians.

VICE PRESIDENT, NURSING: That may be, but the geriatrics center seems to be equally attractive, given the demographics of our population and our competitor's new program. Maybe the geriatric nurse practitioners could be financially involved in some way, too.

CHIEF OPERATING OFFICER: It's not always clear to me what we mean by a joint venture. We could expand space in the clinic for sports medicine, which would certainly result in more admissions and ancillary revenue, but this would not necessarily require an "investment" by the hospital and the physicians.

VICE PRESIDENT, NURSING: We have to approach these opportunities with considerable care. The initial PPO discussions were not well received and there is considerable suspicion about the hospital's motives. Many of our staff could be tempted to invest, but they need to fully understand the risks so that lack of immediate financial success will not sour them completely and damage existing relationships.

PRESIDENT OF MEDICAL STAFF (dropping by the table): What's happening with the PPO proposal? We've stirred up a lot of interest, but there is concern as well. If we don't move ahead there will be a lot of anger, and Suburban Hospital may pick up the initiative. By the way, I heard a speaker at the state medical society meeting who said it's easy to set up something called a MeSH to administer the operation.

CHIEF OPERATING OFFICER: Bill (the CEO) mentioned to me this morning that the vice chair of the board had heard about the laboratory proposal. He was asking if there are legal or ethical issues in referrals to laboratories in which the physician has an ownership interest.

VICE PRESIDENT, PLANNING: There are too many issues, ideas, and recent developments floating around here. We should put everything on hold for six months to decide on an orderly process for considering and operating these projects. If we don't, we are going to get into big trouble and any potential benefits will seem minor in retrospect. We need to clarify the impact of safe harbors and the recent IRS ruling on joint ventures.

CHIEF FINANCIAL OFFICER: That sounds good, but we can't wait— those planning processes always take two or three times longer than intended. We've got two projects that are in the final stages, and we need to decide now to fish or cut bait.

VICE PRESIDENT, MEDICAL AFFAIRS: How do MeSHs work in reality? How can these ventures be structured? Can a single MeSH handle such a broad set of ventures, or are multiple organizations needed?

Physician-Hospital Relationships to Deal with Joint Ventures

Three ways to form physician-hospital relationships were considered by the officers of medical staff and the hospital to deal with the problem of joint venture proposals. One was a committee of the present medical staff organization. The second and third models involved the creation of an outside business corporation that would be jointly owned by physicians and the hospital.

The first alternative, a committee of the organized medical staff, would involve the senior officers of the staff and the chiefs of each of the services. They would meet together, as a venture analysis committee, to review proposals, to initiate proposals, and to put "deals" together. Senior administrators would serve in a staff capacity for the committee. There would be no financial investment in the committee. (Figure 15.1 shows the composition of the committee.)

A second alternative for bringing together physicians and the hospital is a single joint venture corporation. This single legal entity is intended to invest in projects that are mutually beneficial to hospital and physician investors. The projects generally involve equipment and real estate acquisitions, specialized treatment centers, and outreach facilities. The structure of this form of physician-hospital relationship was developed originally by Paul Ellwood and has come to be known as the Medical Staff Hospital (MeSH) model.[1] Figure 15.2 shows a typical MeSH structure. Note the creation of a Venture Analysis Board (VAB), which receives funds and recommends projects for the single enterprise. The projects are shown as joint ventures. Risks, losses, and profits accrue to the Hospital Holding Corporation and the Physician Investment Corporation.

Consultants to the hospital prepared an analysis of the traditional MeSH. They found the single Venture Analysis Board appealing because of its simplicity. More important, however, the consultants criticized the traditional MeSH as unworkable and ineffective for the following reasons:

1. Since most physicians are suspicious and uncertain of the rapid changes in the practice of medicine, they hesitate to invest in the corporation.

2. Not all physicians are prepared to make the substantial investments necessary to allow the MeSH to embark on significant projects.

3. Not all physicians wish to participate in every health care venture.

4. It is difficult to secure physician agreement on investment priorities.

5. The single venture model often subjects the MeSH entity to greater regulation, tax exposure, and significant costs, particularly in the area of securities registration.

Finally, the consultants recommended a third type of joint venture relationship, the modular MeSH, which permits an individualized joint venture for each project, once it has been approved by the hospital-physician corporate group. Figure 15.3 illustrates the features of the modular MeSH.

In the modular MeSH, all prospective ventures under consideration by the hospital would be presented to the Venture Analysis Board.

Figure 15.1 Venture Analysis Committee of an Organized Medical Staff

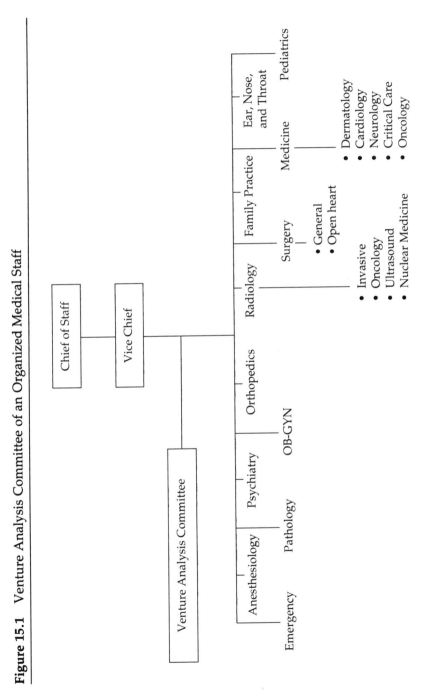

Figure 15.2 Diagram of Traditional MeSH Structure

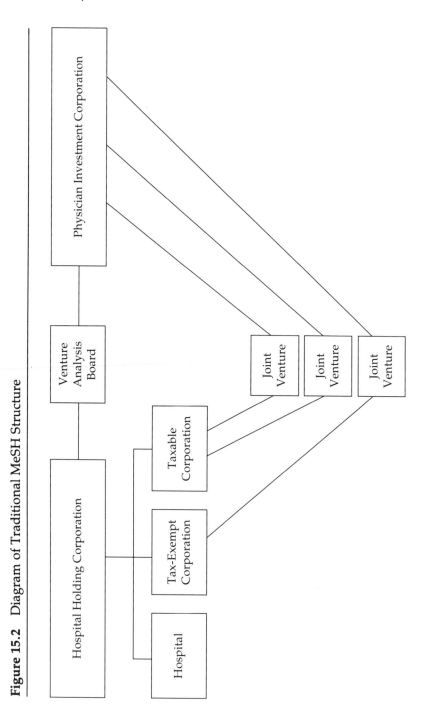

Figure 15.3 Diagram of the Modular MeSH Structure

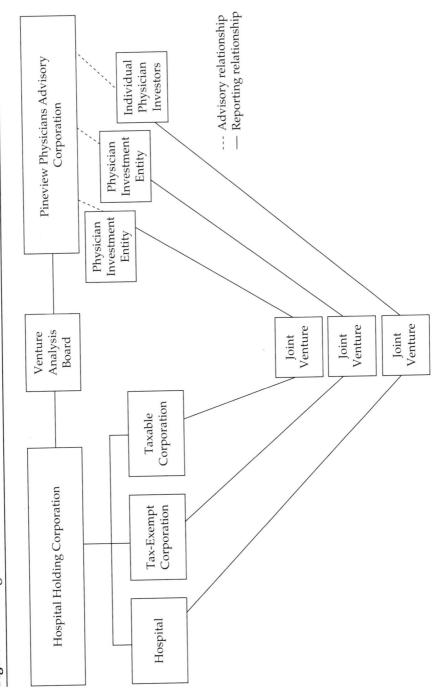

The board would consist of representatives of both the hospital and Pineview Physicians Advisory Corporation (PPAC). The hospital would designate three members to the VAB, usually the chief executive officer, the chief financial officer, and a member of the holding company board of directors. The three PPAC representatives to the VAB should be the president of PPAC, the elected chief of the medical staff (if a member of PPAC), and one other physician who possesses entrepreneurial skills and who would be designated by the board of directors of PPAC.

Once approved by the VAB as worthy of pursuit, the venture would be presented to the PPAC membership. The shareholders of PPAC would have the opportunity to review and question the detailed report of the VAB and exercise an individual choice to participate in any given venture. Neither the membership nor the board of directors of PPAC would have veto power over a PPAC member wishing to participate in a VAB-recommended venture. All members of the medical staff would be encouraged and welcomed to join PPAC and to receive the VAB reports. If members of PPAC were to decide that a given venture is attractive, they would so indicate, and only those members interested in the given venture would proceed to structure the legal and financial relationships for the venture. In other words, members would be given first rights of refusal.

In the event that none of the members of PPAC choose to participate in a joint venture approved by the VAB, the hospital would have the option of proceeding alone or in participation with investors who are not members of PPAC.

Note

1. Paul Ellwood, "The MeSH Model for Hospital-Physicians Joint Venture." Paul Ellwood and Associates, Minneapolis, MN.

Case 16

The Goodbody/LaGrange Merger: What Do You Do When the Judge Says No?

Timothy H. Sio, Robert B. Klint, M.D., and Jerry Rose

Mark Bisbee, M.D., the chief operating officer at Goodbody Hospital, hung up the telephone and sat quietly in his office reflecting on the news he had just received from hospital attorney George Westby. U.S. District Judge Audrey Somewell had decided to disrupt a merger between Goodbody Hospital and LaGrange Medical Center and grant a permanent injunction. It all ended quietly and unceremoniously on a chilly Friday in February, almost three years after Goodbody's president, Robert Hart, M.D., had explored the idea of a hospital merger with community and business leaders and received their support to pursue the concept. Or had he?

On 29 September 1987, the combined boards of LaGrange Corporation and Goodbody Corporation announced the signing of a Memorandum of Understanding that would result in the merger of their two organizations. According to the Hart-Scott-Rodino (HSR) Act of 1976, consolidations, acquisitions, and mergers must be reported to the Federal Trade Commission (FTC) if one component has assets or sales in excess of $100 million and the other has assets of at least $10 million. This notification triggers a premerger timetable during which either the FTC or the U.S. Department of Justice may request further written information. Of 1,400 transactions reported under the HSR Act in 1984, 80 percent were screened out and 20 percent were fully investigated. Second requests for information are occasionally made (i.e., in 5.5 percent of the cases) Mergers are rarely challenged (e.g., 6 of 1,400 were challenged in 1986).

In the case of the Goodbody/LaGrange merger, 72,000 pages of information were reported under HSR in November 1987. Additional information was requested in January 1988 and was provided in February 1988. On 1 June 1988, the U.S. Department of Justice filed a complaint against Goodbody Corporation and LaGrange Corporation in U.S. District Court. The government alleged that the merger would violate Section 7 of the Clayton Antitrust Act and Section 1 of the Sherman Act. The government requested a permanent injunction against the merger. The evidentiary hearing lasted from 20 June to 14 July 1988. The three legal acts affecting this care are described in Appendix 16.1.

On 4 January 1989, Judge Somewell informed counsel from both parties that he had thoroughly reviewed the "Proposed Findings of Fact and Conclusions of Law," would dispense with oral arguments, and expected to render an opinion in the next several weeks.

The Marketplace

The city of Fairview (population 140,000) is located in a county with a population of 251,000 and three relatively large general acute care hospitals. They are LaGrange Medical Center, with 490 beds, Goodbody Hospital, with 427 beds, and Saint Bernadette Hospital, with 303 beds. Each hospital is considered tertiary in its scope of service, and there are significant duplications of services, including three open-heart programs, two linear accelerators, two MRIs, two Level 1 trauma programs, and two pediatric intensive care programs. Relevant utilization data include the following from 1988 data:

	Net Revenue	Occupancy %	Patient Days	Physicians
LaGrange	$ 85.7	73.8	111,626	150
Goodbody	$ 67.0	64.5	92,753	190*
St. Bernadette	$ 51.9	62.7	59,490	100*

*Many physicians have active staff privileges at both.

Two of the three hospitals are in good financial condition, with 1988 net income from operations of $6.9 million at LaGrange, $2.3 million at Goodbody, and a deficit of $7.4 million at Saint Bernadette. Based upon 1988 state-inventoried beds, the hospitals' market shares are as follows: 36 percent for LaGrange, 34 percent for Goodbody, and 25 percent for Saint Bernadette.

Twelve miles to the east, in Millican, a community of about 20,000 in a different county, two additional hospitals rely on Fairview physicians for their specialty care. Because of distance and eco-political connections, they are included in the Fairview standard metropolitan statistical area (SMSA). The two hospitals are St. Mary's, which has 100 beds and 3 percent of the 1988 market share, and Parkview, with 69 beds and 2 percent of the market share. In addition, there are seven contiguous counties in the Fairview SMSA that contain 12 additional hospitals.

LaGrange and Goodbody are 501(c)(3) independent community hospitals. Saint Bernadette is a member of the Third Order of St. Mary's. All three are teaching affiliates of the university's college of medicine.

The major third party payers are Medicare, traditional indemnity insurance, self-insured employers, Medicaid, and HMOs, in that order. For the fiscal years 1987 and 1988, the hospitals received payments from these sources in the following breakdowns:

Fiscal Year 1988

	Medicare	Medicaid	Other
LaGrange	36%	13%	51%
St. Bernadette	44	8	48
Goodbody	37	12	51

Fiscal Year 1987

	Medicare	Medicaid	Other
LaGrange	33%	12%	55%
St. Bernadette	44	7	49
Goodbody	35	9	56

The Merger Process

Prior to the 29 September 1987 merger announcement by the two hospitals, and right up until Judge Somewell's decision, both organizations made significant commitments of time, resources, and money to the merger process. Antitrust regulations prevented the hospitals from discussing any money-making details like operating costs, rates, and medical staff, but there were other important fundamental activities that had to take place if the merger was to be successful. Following exploration of the merger concept and the consensus-building effort by Dr. Hart, there were three distinct phases in the process: information gathering, developing communications management and public relations, and planning implementation strategies.

Information gathering

The hospital CEOs and selected board members visited hospitals that were in the midst of mergers. A merger consultant was also selected and an institutional profile document developed. The profile described the two corporations, summarizing their respective programs, markets, financial performance, resources, medical staffs, and organizational structures. Future plans and strategies were not included. In addition, the consultant developed a key resource document that more specifi-cally detailed the capabilities of the two hospitals with particular empha-sis on people and their talents. In July 1987, a public relations firm was selected to assist the hospitals with the transition needed to make the two organizations into one. This would include the development of a detailed communications plan for key stakeholder groups (physicians, employees, and the community) and the development of a new identity. Legal counsel was also selected to assist in the preparation of docu-ments requested by the Federal Trade Commission and the U.S. Depart-ment of Justice, and to sort out the many legal implications of bringing together two distinctly different multimillion-dollar organizations. Fi-nally, in November 1987, an economic consultant was selected to assist in preparing financial plans, pro formas, and economic rationales.

Developing communications management and public relations

A joint vision statement was drafted by the merger consultant with input from both CEOs. An internal publication, the *Consolidated Review,* was created and a total of eight issues were published to keep key stakeholders informed of the merger progress. A consolidation commit-tee, comprising five board members from each hospital and the two CEOs, was appointed (and was likely to become the new corporation's board of directors). A job opportunities statement was drafted to dem-onstrate growth opportunities for personnel, in an attempt to minimize the anticipated loss of talent. The culmination of this phase was the approval of the Memorandum of Understanding (intent to merge) by both hospital boards and the announcement to employees, the general community, and both medical staffs in September 1987.

Planning implementation strategies

Between November 1987 and June 1988, a number of important implementation strategies were initiated. A planning retreat for executive management and joint boards was held to discuss potential problems, the merger process in general, and key result areas, and to develop a calendar for the integration. A notice of intent was filed with the Federal Trade Commission and the U.S. Department of Justice, and a response to the HSR Act was developed. In late 1987 and late 1988, implementation task forces were named to study the problems of integration, priorities, duplications, and potential efficiencies in the following areas:

— Parent organization and structure
— Name and identity
— Oncology (program integration; physicians participated in the study)
— Laboratory (economics and service issues, if centralized)
— Human resources (salary and benefits issues)
— Transportation (reorganization of helicopter service)
— Trauma (strategy and role in system about to be designated by state)
— Nurses and allied health, recruitment and retention (structure, roles, and strategies)
— School of medicine (integration plan for medical education)
— Wellness programming (eliminate duplicate programs)
— Regional relationships (strategy for garnering support and for benefits to smaller regional hospitals)
— MRI/Lithotripsy (future plans to avoid duplicate services)
— Physician relationships (communications plan, integration of medical staff bylaws and committees)

The findings and recommendations of the task forces were shared with the officers of both organizations. In addition, a retreat with officers, boards, medical staff, and spouses was held to "get to know one another." Letters were sent to members of congress to request their support and explain the purpose. This phase concluded with a retreat featuring a well-known health care futurist, who gave a talk entitled "How to Make Your Merger Work." The consultant's evaluation of the individual corporate cultures was discussed.

Legal Events

In June and July of 1988 the tempo of legal activity accelerated. A response was received from the HSR inquiry and a second submission of requested data was made to the U.S. Department of Justice. On 1 June 1988, the Justice Department filed a complaint against LaGrange and Goodbody Corporations and requested a preliminary injunction. The issue was debated in late June and July. After 20 days and 21 witnesses, the hearing ended. What follows are extracts from the "Proposed Findings of Fact and Conclusions of Law" that were submitted by both parties at the conclusion of the evidentiary trial. They illustrate the different interpretations of the facts and the arguments used by both sides in the case.

United States	*Goodbody/LaGrange*
Both hospitals are involved in interstate commerce. A not-for-profit status is irrelevant because research shows they act like for-profits in exercising market power.	The Department of Justice has no jurisdiction over the merger of not-for-profit hospitals because stocks and assets are neither purchased nor traded as specified in Section 7 of the Clayton Act. The FTC Act itself acknowledges its limited jurisdiction over not-for-profits.
Both hospitals are financially sound.	Both hospitals are at risk and are experiencing declining financial strength because of prospective payment, charity, and declining utilization.
Acute inpatient care is the relevant product market.	All patient care is the relevant product market.
• There is no substitute of diagnosis or treatment when a doctor determines it is necessary.	• Outpatient centers compete for patients with hospitals.
• The State distinguishes inpatient from outpatient care in its contracting.	• The hospital can substitute outpatient care and there is cross-elasticity of demand.

- The merger does not include psychiatric substance abuse and inpatient rehab because they represent a different kind of care.
- Acute inpatient care is the most common product offered. It is more important to cost, and it nets the highest proportion of revenues.

The Fairview area is the relevant geographic market

- Patients and doctors prefer to use hospitals that are close to them.

- Doctors outside Fairview are not on Fairview hospital staffs.
- Fairview residents do not migrate out; 93 percent receive all care in the area.
- Ninety percent of all patients in the two hospitals come from only five counties.

- The hospitals compete only with one another.
- Other administrators in the area testified that they don't compete with Fairview.

New entries into the product market are very unlikely because of cost, excess capacity, and certificate-of-need laws.

- Payers limit payments for inpatient care.

- Outpatient business is 20 percent of total and increasing. St. Bernadette is part of a strong and competitive eight-hospital system that would be unaffected by the merger.

The hospitals serve a ten-county area in a 25-mile radius.

- The government's data are flawed: only phone interviews were used, the method was not scientific, and other data were ignored.
- Patients migrate into Fairview for care.
- St. Bernadette admits to being a "regional center."

- Other administrators, including several from surrounding metropolitan areas, testified that they compete with Fairview.
- A high percentage of patients come to Fairview for care.
- The Elzenga-Hogarty test establishes relevant geographic markets by determining where migration out is minimal (less than 10 percent) and migration in is minimal. It shows that the market includes at least 10 counties.

St. Bernadette (and others) can increase availability of beds because they don't now use all their licensed beds.

The Case

Goodbody Hospital has 60 days to appeal Judge Somewell's ruling. If his decision stands, this will be the first time the government has successfully blocked the merger of two not-for-profit hospitals. This decision could have a significant impact on similar cases nationwide. Consolidations, acquisitions, and mergers are increasing in frequency. There are estimates that 60 percent of not-for-profit, nongovernmental hospitals will be part of a system by 1995. Because of excess capacity, operating deficits, lower margins, and high capital costs, 700 hospitals are expected to close by 1995.

LaGrange and Goodbody combined have more than 900 beds, total expenditures of $140 million a year, and more than 3,500 employees. The merger was projected to result in a $40 million savings over five years and a facility that would become a first-class regional tertiary care center, rivaling those in nearby states. Increased capital resources and volume of patients would allow more specialized care, including organ transplants. Total direct cost to the two corporations to date for legal, consulting, and related merger activities is $1.8 million. The cost to the government is unknown. There is a lot at stake. Will Dr. Hart and Goodbody file the appeal?

Appendix 16.1: The Laws

The Sherman Act (1890) was a congressional response to growing public dissatisfaction with industrial monopolies. It is considered the Magna Carta of antitrust laws. Section I prohibits contracts and combinations that restrain trade. It applies to not-for-profit and for-profit organizations and addresses restraint actions that have already been taken.

The Clayton Act (1914) was passed at President Wilson's request because of failures to control the growth of monopolies through the Sherman Act. It is now the government's primary weapon against mergers and monopolies. Section 7 prohibits the acquisition of stocks or assets when such action will lead to substantial reductions in competition in the future. The *U.S. v. Philadelphia Bank* case (1963) extended the scope of jurisdiction to include the "exchange" of stock as well as acquisition. Companies that are privately held also fall within Clayton's scope following the *U.S. v. Chelsea Savings Bank* case (1969).

The Hart-Scott-Rodino Act (1976) specifies which transactions must be reported to the Federal Trade Commission and what procedures will be followed for review of information.

Part VI

Accountability

Leadership and Social Responsibility

Martin Cherkasky, M.D.

In practice it is seldom very hard to do one's duty when one knows what it is, but it is sometimes exceedingly difficult to find this out.

—Samuel Butler, "First Principles," *Note Books* (1912)

In the golden years of American medicine immediately after World War II, when both physicians and patients were comfortable with the informal social contract of compassion on one side and trust on the other, the possibilities of treatment constantly expanded, as did the number of people who had access to that treatment. This success brought about many of today's painful dilemmas, as the potential of medicine increased geometrically and the expectations of individual patients kept pace. A general belief developed that medical care was a universal right, but the nation never reached a consensus about the commitment of resources necessary to implement that right.

This growing conflict was given an explosive impetus with the Social Security Amendments of 1965, which established Medicare and Medicaid and poured billions of dollars into the health care industry. The organized medical profession was so opposed to this powerful social legislation that little thought was given to the possible consequences of the great infusion of money into the system. The medical leadership abdicated its responsibility to reassure the public that it would not only protect the legitimate interests of physicians but would collectively protect the interests of the population. The actions of organized medicine in fighting the passage of Medicare legislation, and since then in resisting regulations, whether good or bad, have convinced many that protection of economic opportunity for physicians has overshadowed other important interests. In this last decade of the twentieth century, when every indication is that there will be more, not less, involvement of outside forces in the delivery of medical care, a fundamental responsibility of physician managers is to convince their colleagues of the ultimate futility of this negative resistance and to involve them positively in the redesign of the relationship of medicine and society.

The time has long passed when physicians alone decide how health care should be managed and delivered and funded. Today, providers, consumers, and purchasers of care, as well as governments, have legitimate and powerful interests and capabilities with regard to the organization, management, and financing of health care. Although the design of the U.S. health care system in the twenty-first century is not yet readily discernible, the fact that there will be many players in addition to physicians has already been settled.

What has not been decided is whether the transition will be accomplished in an atmosphere of collaboration or of conflict. If the physician leader looks at all that has happened and decides that the physician is a victim, mirroring the attitude of many groups of doctors, then we are headed toward more confrontation, a further withering of the physician's status in the community, the turning away of the country's best and brightest from medicine, and a worsening outlook for both practitioners and patients in the United States.

These changed circumstances place new burdens on physician executives. No longer can they afford to behave like union leaders who fight solely for the welfare of their workers. New managerial responsibilities require that while executives must protect the doctors' legitimate interests, they must also move away from the rhetoric that says that only doctors are concerned with the welfare of patients. Tough decisions about health care organization, management, and financing must not be made into tests of strength between opposing sides. Physician executives must recognize that these are public decisions about the public welfare, and that in a democratic society they are made in the political arena. The first test of accountability for physician executives should be their ability to develop in their physicians better understanding of these complicated issues, to bring about their participation in a dialogue with respect for the appropriate interest of the community and the government in health care.

Such discussions, and solutions for the questions raised, require an awareness of competing interests, of the necessity of balancing worthy but differing claims on resources. Accountability for leadership in such difficult areas includes responsibility where there is no clear-cut right or wrong; where there are multiple views about what should or could be done; where outcomes at times leave everybody dissatisfied. These issues are far more complicated than relatively simple questions such as whether patients are seen in a timely fashion, whether the books are balanced, and whether the facility is neat and clean. Higher levels of performance are required and accountability takes on a different meaning for the physician manager.

The Physician Executive

In many enterprises, the manager is someone with a particular expertise related to the company's basic processes. Being a physician represents extraordinary education and experience. In health care, the manager who is also a physician offers an important advantage to the institution: the capacity to understand physicians and their craft. Both in internal management and in external relationships, the cachet provided by the physician's qualifications is often a powerful tool.

The first duty of every manager is to insure the viability of the enterprise. No dreams of great public service or succoring the sick are meaningful if financial or operational failure occurs. In addition, physician executives have other goals: to handle money and personnel effectively; to attract and keep clients, skilled physicians, and good employees; to be able to acquire the best equipment; to keep the facility clean and safe. They look forward to growth, improvement, and better services. They strive to establish a reputation that brings in patients and draws favorable community attention. They want everything about their organizations to stand for quality and compassion, to provide good care for patients and a good working environment for employees.

Similar managerial goals are found in every complex undertaking. But, while this kind of accountability suffices for most commercial business, there is more required of executives in medical and health care enterprises. Care for the sick and the prevention of illness are primarily moral activities. The essential nobility involved in one human being caring for another is in many ways the definition of humanity. The fear of illness, impairment, handicap, and death is a universal reality, and has led to laws that prevent anyone from denying the sick access to care.

There is an underlying and powerful pact between medicine, the healing professions, and society. Health care is a special activity that the public supports in an extraordinarily generous manner, providing trillions of dollars to build schools of medicine, nursing, and dentistry, as well as research labs, hospitals, and clinics. Society gives physicians a special status. Even today, when dissatisfaction with health care and the questioning of doctors' methods are widespread, individual Americans may have doubts about doctors in general, but they still believe that their own doctors are special and devoted to their interests. Because health care has this kind of meaning to society as a whole, representing a shield against the most ubiquitous threat to patients and their families; because the capacity of medicine to cure and heal moves ahead by leaps and bounds; because this remarkable boon is organized and financed in a way that makes it difficult and costly, or impossible to get—for all of these reasons, there is inevitably the kind of communal, public, and political involvement in health care that we see in the United States today. On every issue, we see a struggle for common ground between a profession that at one time set all the rules about medicine and health care with public approval, and the public, which now wants to help make decisions. Today the physician executive must fulfill the endless series of tasks and responsibilities needed to make organizations run well. The physician executive and the governing body must continually count among their most pressing responsibilities a productive response to the community's views, wishes, and needs.

Medicine and Society

In a democracy, "the government" is not an alien force but the creation of the people, so it must be open to influence and pressure. Perhaps the most important responsibility of every physician executive manager is to work in all local, state, and national areas where public policy is made, in an effort to bring the resources of society fully to bear on problems that can only be resolved through a massive social effort. Are we to sit quietly by while, despite the fact that we spend more of our gross national product on health care than any other nation, we remain the only democracy (or developed country, for that matter) that leaves such a large percentage of its people (37 million at last count) without health care coverage?

The managers of health care resources are stewards of a powerful and magnificent product of human ingenuity. One of our chief responsibilities, despite preoccupation with the survival of our own enterprise, is to constantly push forward the frontiers of service and concern for the society we serve. Our present health care system is expensive, inefficient, and clumsily regulated. To make the juggernaut more compassionate, more effective, and more affordable, and directed by a less burdensome regulatory machine, we will need the active participation of those most knowledgeable about medical care and its delivery. Today's physician executives will be held accountable by their successors and by tomorrow's patients for their role in this process.

The Part VI Cases

The three cases in Part VI all relate to the physician executive's accountability to the community and to his or her ability to involve other physicians in developing solutions to quasi-political problems.

The three cases also illustrate that political skills and a knowledge of the political process are essential to the modern physician executive and that the barriers erected in medicine between various categories of patients or institutions are essentially artificial. Once care for one class of patient is regulated, all are affected. If certain standards are set for Medicare clients, other patients in the same hospital will be treated and discharged according to the same criteria. All the physicians in the state medical society, no matter who their patients, have an interest in the malpractice law. The HMOs will develop practice standards that apply to all patients, not just the Medicaid patients. Although public hospitals carry a greater burden of social problems such as the boarder babies, all the hospitals in a big city are affected when social difficulties such as poverty, homelessness, and drug addiction increase.

Malpractice and the state medical society

The cost of malpractice insurance, the subject of the first case, is a heavy weight upon individual physicians and upon particular specialties, regions, and hospitals. It is a significant factor in the intolerably and rapidly rising cost of health care in the whole country. Any administrator who hopes to affect the laws around this difficult subject will need a high level of political skill and a sound knowledge of the law and of the intricacies of medical practice. The role of the leader of a state medical society or any other physician organization is not to encourage the natural anxieties of the members but to help them understand underlying issues and work toward possible solutions.

The president of the medical society is aware of the degree of emotion that will be pervasive in the room when he returns from the break in the meeting. He knows how upset, angry, and annoyed some of his colleagues are about the malpractice crisis. He has heard cries for action from both ends of the spectrum, from those who wish to refuse to deliver the offspring of lawyers, and from those of a less vengeful temperament. The president has three broad responsibilities: (1) to maintain the medical society as a unified group that is capable of representing the physicians of the state in this and future dealings with the authorities and the community; (2) to recognize the reality of the psychic and financial pain endured by some members and persuade them to stay the course; and (3) to propose steps that hold promise for resolving the issue in an equitable fashion in the foreseeable future.

Case questions

1. What are Dr. Finnegan's options?
2. Should he use his party affiliation to help the society? How could he do this?
3. Why was the society successful in the Senate and unsuccessful in the House?
4. Can you suggest better or different lobbying strategies?
5. What can Dr. Finnegan learn from the state trial lawyer's association?
6. How should Dr. Finnegan try to unify his membership? Is it possible?

Medicaid, HMOs, and quality assurance

Dr. Bergan, the medical director of the HMO, is caught between two irreconcilable interests on the part of the state. The first is cost containment. The state mandated the enrollment of Medicaid recipients in HMOs, with the promise to the taxpayers that dollars would be saved. At the same time, the state wants assurance that the care given to Medicaid recipients is of reasonable quality. Health care, like other commodities, is always delivered in accordance with the pattern set by financial arrangements. Instead of recognizing this fundamental proposition, the purchasers of care frequently set up the rules in accordance with their own financial priorities and then attempt by restrictions, supervision, audits, and penalties to produce an outcome that does not flow naturally from the system of funding. In a prepaid, capitation system of reimbursement, there is already pressure to underutilize services, a reluctance or even a refusal to provide services, and rationing of the more expensive services. A demand for quality assurance is likely to be seen as one more unnecessary burden.

Case questions

1. Is it possible for Dr. Bergan to keep both the state and the individual physicians happy?
2. Must quality be sacrificed to save money?
3. What choices are available to Dr. Bergan?
4. Why are the physicians resistant to a quality assurance program?

5. How can Dr. Bergan involve the physicians in the design of the quality assurance program?

6. How can he find allies to help in negotiations with the state?

Boarder babies

The Metropole Health and Hospitals Corporation, with 16 hospitals and over 10,000 beds, houses at any time around 200 babies who have completed inpatient treatment but have remained unclaimed by any family member. Because suitable foster care is unavailable in a city where the number of children in foster care has doubled in five years, they stay as inpatients for months and even years. There is general agreement that this is bad for the babies and a waste of desperately needed hospital resources. Every president of the corporation faces this problem, and every one fails to find a solution.

Despite Metropole's financial problems, the city's 1990 budget is over $27 billion, larger than that of many independent nations. The Health and Hospitals Corporation's budget is over $2.5 billion.

The "boarder babies" are akin to the thousands of homeless people on the streets of the city, the thousands of other children for whom the city agencies cannot find appropriate foster care, and all the other dependent people for whom the city struggles unsuccessfully to provide. Boarder babies are just one of the terrible social ills for which the city and the nation have not found a solution.

By virtue of her position as the head of one of the largest undertakings in the city, which delivers one of the most important and fundamental services in the city and interacts with so many other city and state agencies, Dr. Paula Valdez has the power and prestige to speak out on behalf of the boarder babies. This kind of social activism and marshaling of public resources is the function of any physician executive who occupies a seat of power. However, she cannot solve the issue by using the overburdened resources of the hospital system.

Case questions

1. What are the political implications that Dr. Valdez must consider?

2. How are public hospitals different from private hospitals?

3. Could this problem be handled within HHC alone?

4. How should Dr. Valdez handle the press?

5. What are Dr. Valdez's immediate, short-term, and long-term strategies?

6. Can social problems such as the boarder babies be solved without a reordering of priorities in local and national spending?

Malpractice and the State Medical Society

Earl R. Thayer

Thomas Finnegan, M.D., a radiologist, is the president of a 6,000-member state medical society. He served for five years on its board of directors and on several committees before becoming president-elect. His term as president is for one year, but as the immediate past president he will serve for another year on the board. He is known as a thoughtful, aggressive, articulate physician. Well regarded as a clinician, he is also politically active, usually voting Democratic but occasionally as an independent.

The medical liability (malpractice) issue has heated up during his presidency. The society's members want a remedy for skyrocketing premium costs, higher frequency of suits, and dramatically increased settlements or jury awards. Many members are militant, threatening to stop work unless something is done quickly. Others say they'll resign their memberships ($450 in dues per year) if the society can't bring relief to their needs. To complicate matters, there is sharp division among the members on how to solve the problem. Most legislators view the matter as a doctors-versus-lawyers issue. The key legislative committee on insurance is chaired by a plaintiff attorney, who vows that no bill that does what the physician wants will ever get out of his committee.

Dr. Finnegan wants to be a good leader, but what should he do and how should he do it?

Background

In 1975, the state legislature, responding to new doctors' inability to obtain insurance coverage from any source and greatly increased premium costs, passed a medical liability bill with five major provisions:

1. All licensed physicians practicing in the state were required to carry professional liability (malpractice) insurance in the minimum amount of $200,000 for one event and $600,000 for all events in any one year. This is called 200/600 coverage, and it could be purchased by the physician from any insurance company willing to write the policy.

2. As a trade-off for the mandated insurance, the legislature set up a patients' compensation fund (PCF) to pay any settlements or jury awards that exceeded the physicians' 200/600 base coverage. There would be no limit on how much could be paid from the PCF for a single malpractice case. The PCF would be operated by the state insurance department and a broadly based board of governors that included representatives of the medical society. All physicians would be required to pay annual assessments into the PCF to ensure that enough money was available to pay such claims.

3. A health care liability insurance plan (HCLIP) was created to be operated by the insurance commissioner and the board of governors to provide 200/600 liability coverage to any physician unable to obtain such protection in the private market. Any physician who applied for coverage was to be accepted at the usual premium rate for his or her classification.

4. A patients' compensation panel program was established, to be administered by the state court system, to provide three-person panels (one lawyer, one physician, one public member) to handle cases up to $10,000 and five-person panels (one lawyer, two MDs, and two public members) to handle claims beyond $10,000. Every person making a malpractice claim was required to file their claim with a panel, which would hear the evidence from both sides, render an opinion, and make awards or settlements. The panel decisions could be appealed to a jury trial in a district court.

5. Whenever a patients' compensation panel found a physician negligent in care of a patient (guilty of malpractice), that finding was to be reported to the state medical examining board for possible discipline.

The Situation

The new system had been operating for ten years, long enough for the "long tail" of medical liability claims to have taken full effect. For a time, the liability problem of availability and cost abated, but now another crisis loomed. The commissioner of insurance, after completing a study, declared that "this crisis is caused by the same components that caused the mid-1970s crisis—only magnified." Skyrocketing premium costs were being passed on to patients in the form of higher charges; physicians were practicing more defensive medicine (also raising patient costs); and health care providers were curtailing or ceasing practice, particularly obstetrics and gynecology, orthopedics, and neurosurgery.

The state medical society board of directors considered this issue thoroughly and made the following proposals to remedy the situation:

1. Require all paid claims involving the death of a patient or settlement for more than $25,000 to be referred to the state medical examining board for possible discipline, and continue to refer all negligence findings by panels. Because 47 percent of all panel cases were settled before the hearing without a finding of negligence, the physicians in almost half the malpractice cases avoided the peer review thought to be built into the system.

2. Limit the dollar amount of award in any malpractice case to no more than $250,000 per occurrence. Seventeen states had adopted some version of a cap on awards ranging from $200,000 to $500,000. Through the use of annuities, an award of $250,000 would produce nearly $1.5 million in benefit over an expected life span, thus fairly treating the claimants. Such a limit would inject a degree of predictability in the system, which would stabilize premium rates.

3. Pay fund settlements or awards on a periodic basis rather than in lump sums. The 1975 law provided that all claims over $1 million be paid in installments of not more than $500,000 per year and that future medical expenses over $25,000 be paid as incurred. The latter was good; the former created windfalls for relatives of injured patients who died, and it did not "match compensation with loss," one of the fund's goals.

4. Require a sliding scale of contingency fees for plaintiff attorneys. Malpractice claims were usually handled by attorneys on a contingency fee basis. The attorney was paid for his or her efforts only if the plaintiff won money. The usual contingency

fee was 33¹/₃ percent of the award or settlement. In some cases, this produced what some felt was an unconscionable reimbursement to the attorney. Attorneys felt that the contingency fee arrangement permitted the poor person access to justice.

5. Require those who file malpractice claims to submit a certificate of merit in each case to certify that the claim was reviewed by a qualified expert and found to be meritorious. Experience showed that 31 percent of all panel cases were dismissed for lack of merit, thus needlessly congesting the system and draining administrative costs.

6. Adopt a collateral source rule to prohibit duplication of benefits. Winning malpractice claimants collected medical expenses from their health, auto, or worker compensation insurance, which duplicated benefits from their malpractice suit. This had a major impact on the cost of medical liability insurance.

7. Limit pain and suffering to $100,000.

The state medical society also had a special liability committee studying the entire issue. It supported, but had not yet put into legislation, the following proposals:

— Reduce the general statute of limitations from three years to two years.

— Increase protection for liability for physicians who participate in peer review.

— Provide for bifurcated trials at panels or in juries, so that determination of negligence and awards would be separate actions.

— Require that losing parties at the panel level post bond of $10,000 if they wish to pursue the case in a jury trial.

— Require insurers to obtain the consent of the insured prior to settlement of a claim.

The society studies also showed that

— the panel system established in 1975 had a very high percentage (27 percent) of nonmeritorious claims;

— the goals of speedy resolution and lower attorney and administrative costs were not being met;

— the panels resulted in an equal percentage of cases winning money for plaintiffs and cases in which physicians were found innocent;

— in the prior jury system and in other states without formal panels, the ratio was 70 to 30 in favor of physicians; and

— the trend was toward all severe claims being appealed to jury trial so that a double trial system was developing with concomitant double costs, time lost, emotional trauma, and jeopardy.

At its annual meeting, the society's delegates from every county agreed to seek passage of a bill (like Senate Bill 100, described below) and to support a nonbinding mediation system as an alternative to the panel system. The medical society participated actively in a special legislative committee along with legislators, attorneys, and other citizens and produced a bill (Senate Bill 100) that was passed by the state senate on 10 April by a vote of 26 to 6. The main provisions of the bill were as follows:

1. Medical malpractice awards limited to $1 million for *nonmedical* expenses with no limit on medical expenses. Of the $1 million, the amount for pain and suffering was limited to $250,000.
2. Medical expenses defined to eliminate costs of housing repairs and unusual educational costs. Medical expenses over $50,000 were to be paid only as incurred. Attorneys were not allowed to take a contingency fee on medical expenses in excess of $50,000.
3. The PCF would set up surcharges for physicians based on actual claims experience.
4. PCF assessments limited to no more than 200 percent of the actual claims paid for the preceding year.
5. An optional nonbinding mediation system would be established to resolve malpractice claims rather than going through the panel system.
6. Any loss or reduction of a physician's hospital staff privileges was to be reported to the medical examining board, and the board at any time in its reasonable judgment could require a physician to submit to a physical, mental, or professional competency examination.

In response, the state trial lawyer's association, dominated by plaintiff attorneys (of which there were about 150), opposed the state medical society's proposals and Senate Bill 100, stating the following:

1. The cap was too low. It should be no lower than $3.3 million.
2. There was no medical malpractice insurance crisis, just the doctors and insurance companies "crying wolf."

3. Medical liability premiums were less than 0.5 percent of all health care costs, and this percentage was declining, not increasing. Thus, the cost was "small per citizen per year."
4. The average doctor paid on 2.9 percent of gross income per year for malpractice insurance, and from 1977 to 1981 the average premium actually declined by 6.5 percent.
5. The cause of malpractice litigation was medical negligence.
6. No limits should be placed on awards for pain and suffering; they were "needed compensation."
7. Government restrictions on attorney's fees were "unfair and would deprive plaintiffs of their rights to sue."

While Senate Bill 100 was not totally acceptable to the state medical society, Dr. Finnegan considered it a reasonable compromise and argued in the legislature for its passage. The full weight of the society's lobbying resources was put into action. The Senate passed Senate Bill 100 by a wide margin. In the House, however, the chair of the insurance committee (a plaintiff attorney and Democrat) to which the Senate-passed bill was referred vowed it would "never see the light of day again." Attempts by the House to override his control of the committee and bring the bill to the floor failed on a party-line vote. The legislature then adjourned for the year, thus effectively eliminating any legislative relief to the malpractice issue for another 12 to 18 months.

Dr. Finnegan perceived the members of his organization to be deeply disappointed in the legislature's failure to enact remedial measures to their malpractice concerns. This was in part a reflection on his leadership abilities. Now the grumbling of members grew louder. There were threats of resignation. More obstetricians quit the practice of deliveries, especially in rural areas. Questions grew about the society's legislative effectiveness. Requests were made for the state society to support work stoppages in all but emergency cases. Calls to boycott attorneys were received. Divisiveness continued over what to do to ease the premium burden and growing number and severity of malpractice claims.

At a quarterly meeting of the board of directors the next month, the following comments were made about the situation:

DR. MUELLER: I can't believe how the legislature could be this irresponsible. It is certainly going to come back to haunt them. Many more physicians will stop performing high-risk cases over the next 18 months, and the system will begin to break down. We will get a bill that is even stronger than Senate Bill 100 in the next session. I think we should drop out of the debate for the next 18 months and let things really heat up.

Dr. KELLY: I agree that we will be in a stronger position in the future, but we need to work actively with the legislature in the coming year. If we do nothing, the trial lawyers' position will be strengthened without a counterposition. I wasn't very happy about the bill myself, and I'd like to start making changes now. Let's appoint a new task force to begin drafting next year's proposal.

Dr. GOLDHAMMER: I can't believe what I am hearing from you guys. This is the most important issue that we have faced in a decade. The members are really hurting, and the credibility of the society is at stake. If we do nothing or appoint another committee, we will look weak and ineffective. I think we should march on the state capitol like they did in Michigan to demonstrate to the legislature and our members that we can act and generate public support.

Dr. COLLINS: I agree with action. Some of my colleagues have suggested "work actions," such as withholding services except for emergencies. And I heard in another state that all the obstetricians have refused to deliver lawyers' babies; that doesn't seem to be an unreasonable action.

Dr. KELLY: We have to be very careful with such suggestions. Patients don't like to see us in political roles, and such actions could lose us the legislative support we have carefully won.

Dr. WARNER: Maybe we could get the governor to call a special session of the legislature next month to deal with this issue alone. I don't think we can wait for 18 months for resolution of this issue.

Dr. GOLDHAMMER: He would never do it; he's a lawyer and a Democrat and has to run for re-election next year. Trying to get doctors and lawyers together is a "no win" for him until after the election.

Dr. KELLY: I have to reluctantly agree. As bad as it is, the issue is too hot to reconsider now, and it will be easier to resolve in a year. Remember, we want to improve on Senate Bill 100, not compromise more.

Dr. COLLINS: I can't believe this discussion. I know that our county group will be furious and maybe do something on their own if we don't do something forceful now.

Dr. Finnegan called for a 30-minute break in the meeting and took a brief walk by the lake. When the meeting reconvened, he would have to recommend an action that the society should take and provide the leadership for this action in the board.

Medicaid, HMOs, and Quality Assurance

Carol Winkler Schramm and Richard M. Carr, M.D.

A news article in April 1981 read as follows:

> A major state budget crisis loomed today amid reports that Medicaid spending is skyrocketing. The governor stated, "Medicaid is out of control and could chew up everything else." The state is likely to begin eliminating some Medicaid benefits as soon as possible, according to the governor's office.

At the same time, the state, a major purchaser of health care, was studying ways to contain employee health care costs. Financial incentives were offered to employees to enroll in HMOs. This strategy was successful, with 67 percent of state employees enrolling in an HMO (compared with a predicted 50 percent). The state employees' health care was provided through the HMO with the most competitive bid. Due to the success of enrollment, the state agency that administered the Medicaid program began studying how HMOs could be used in the Medicaid delivery system.

When Medicaid spending was compared to the cost of health care for state employees, it was estimated that coverage costing $119 million a year could be provided for $95.5 million (projected savings of $23.5 million) if Medicaid recipients were enrolled in HMOs. The federal Health Care Financing Administration was asked for a waiver of the freedom-of-choice provision of the Medicaid program. In 1983, the

Medicaid agency received this waiver, which allowed mandatory enrollment of Medicaid recipients in HMOs in two of the larger counties of
the state. Medicaid recipients had to enroll in an HMO, but they could
choose which of the participating HMOs they wanted to enroll in.

This program, known as the mandatory enrollment initiative
(MEI), began in Adams County in July 1984 and in Brown County in
October 1984. The 13 HMOs joining the MEI were for-profit, nationally
owned organizations and nonprofit, locally organized groups arising
out of community clinics and health centers. Table 18.1 provides data
on the HMOs participating in the MEI.

For many HMOs in Brown County, participation in the MEI was
a necessity, not an option. Medicaid recipients constituted a large part
of the patient base (one out of every six). To protect this base, four new
HMOs were formed as a direct result of the initiative. Even though the
capitation rate was discounted by 7 percent from the preexisting fee-for-
service utilization figures, there was a lot of "fat" in the system and
substantial earnings could be made.

The number of patient days per 1,000 enrollee years in Brown
County prior to the initiative was 1,198 in 1983 and 1,044 in 1984; this
was for a relatively young and healthy population of mothers and children. After a year of HMO involvement, this figure dropped to 461 days
per 1,000 (1985), a 56 percent decrease. By 1986, the figure had dropped
to 354 days per 1,000. Length of stay dropped from an average of 5.9 to
3.4 days, and admissions fell from 208 to 129 per 1,000. During the first
year, ambulance and emergency room use was cut in half. Physician
visits also dropped from 4.4 per enrollee in 1984 to 3.3 per enrollee in
1985. Utilization of prescriptions and laboratory and x-ray examinations
increased. The net result was some initial savings for the Medicaid
program and income for the HMOs, especially those with large numbers
of enrollees. Some larger Medicaid-dominated HMOs with good control
programs were able to pay off start-up loans and accumulate reserves
of up to $1 million in a two-year period.

An additional financial advantage to participate in the initiative
was that enrollees were capitated on an individual basis; there were no
family rates. Even though the individual rate was lower for Medicaid
enrollees, $65 versus $90 for commercial enrollees, the HMO made up
this difference by using only single capitation rates. For example, the
HMO received $260 per month (4 × $65) for a family of four on Medicaid and $220 per month for a family of four for commercial enrollees.
Thus, Medicaid paid $260 per month for a family with only one adult,
and the commercials paid $220 per month for a family with two adults.
This difference helped to offset the lower Medicaid rate. Government

Table 18.1 HMOs in the Mandatory Enrollment Initiative, January 1987

Model	Type	Total Enrollment	1/1/87 Total Medicaid Enrollment	Percent of Medicaid Enrollment	1986 Medicaid Payment (in millions)	Total Age in Years	Number of MDs	Number of Primary Care Physicians
A Staff	Cooperative	54,009	1,529	3.0%	1.1	8.0	NK	38 FTE
B Staff	Cooperative	38,600	2,157	5.6	1.3	11.0	NK	19 FTE
C Clinic	For-profit	73,000	4,166	5.6	2.3	2.9	600	111
D Clinic	For-profit	51,366	3,585	7.0	2.0	0.6	298	166
E Clinic	Nonprofit	13,000	13,000	100.0	9.3	2.7	270	13 FTE
F IPA	For-profit	6,000	3,176	53.0	2.4	2.0	288	126
G IPA	For-profit	27,017	572	2.1	0.3	3.7	1,836	181
H IPA	For-profit	11,286	11,286	NK	9.3	2.5	170	98
I IPA	For-profit	190,000	13,067	7.0	8.2	8.0	NK	NK
J IPA	For-profit	37,646	17,274	46.0	12.7	1.8	1,189	NK
Medqual	For-profit	44,000	22,000	50.0	19.3	3.0	1,100	450
K IPA	For-profit	30,523	12,571	41.0	11.5	1.0	1,050	464
Healthrite	For-profit	81,000	16,500	20.3	14.3	4.8	760	240

Note: NK = Not known; FTE = Full-time equivalent, not a count of actual number of physicians.

payments often were delayed, but the financial benefits outweighed, or at least balanced, the negative aspects.

The mandatory nature of the program and the relatively rapid development of HMOs for the financing and delivery of health care services to Medicaid recipients made it essential that quality, access, and satisfaction be examined carefully. Because the state received a waiver of the federal freedom-of-choice requirement, Medicaid recipients lost the ability to move freely among providers. To counteract this, the state stipulated that all HMOs delivering medical care to Medicaid enrollees have a quality assurance (QA) program as an integral part of their organization.

The HMOs had different attitudes concerning their responsibility to provide adequate QA. The state had not provided specific funds for development of a QA Program. Some HMOs viewed QA as a concern of the medical organization with which it contracted to deliver health care (i.e., IPAs and hospitals). Some HMO administrators also felt that since the state had licensing power and a certification program for Medicaid providers, it should bear the burden for maintaining quality among providers.

The HMO administrative budgets varied from 8 percent to 13 percent of the premium dollar, a figure that administrators felt could not go higher. Some HMOs saw utilization review (UR) as a reasonable substitute for QA; however, the state mandate stipulated that QA issues must be separated from UR considerations.

Smaller HMOs faced resource limitations, although they were committed to delivering a high-quality product to their enrollees, while some larger HMOs had adequate resources but faced philosophical limitations. All HMOs were concerned about provider response to implementation of a monitoring system with the goal of improved quality of care.

Healthrite HMO

Healthrite HMO is located in Watertown, the county seat of Brown County. The population of Brown County is 900,000, with 750,000 residing in Watertown. This is a heterogeneous population with approximately 120,000 urban poor who are eligible for Aid to Families with Dependent Children (AFDC) and Medicaid. Roughly one in every six persons is a Medicaid recipient. Healthrite is a network-model HMO with nine independent practice associations (IPAs). In five years, Healthrite has grown from 19,000 to over 81,000 enrollees. It contracts with four general hospitals and one specialty hospital. There are over

760 physicians in the nine IPAs—240 primary care physicians and 520 specialists.

As the medical director of Healthrite Dr. Bergan is in charge of the UR and QA programs. He supervises a QA and UR manager who has a staff of five nurses. The QA and UR programs consist primarily of inpatient chart reviews and deal with individual quality concerns identified through the UR process. Dr. Bergan is an internist who has practiced medicine for 17 years, the last 12 in a multispeciality clinic in Watertown. He served on the board of Service Corporation and has been a member of the hospital peer review committee. Four years ago, his clinic joined Healthrite HMO. Shortly after joining, he was asked to serve on the UR committee. He served on that committee for two years before taking his current half-time position as Healthrite Corporate Medical Director.

In October of 1984, Healthrite HMO entered into a contract with the state Medicaid agency to provide care on a capitated basis for 16,500 AFDC Medicaid recipients (20 percent of the total enrollees) who enrolled between November 1984 and February 1985. When Dr. Bergan became the medical director, the transfer of these recipients into the HMO was almost complete. Dr. Bergan had not been involved in the negotiation process on the Medicaid contract. When he became the medical director, he faced a situation in which the HMO was overwhelmed by the rapid influx of the Medicaid population. The HMO administrative system had to enroll the recipients, assign primary care physicians, and educate enrollees about the Healthrite provider network and use of the HMO system. Instituting utilization controls and reviews for these new enrollees was a major task. In addition, four new provider groups joined Healthrite HMO in late 1984, so Dr. Bergan was dealing with over 320 new providers. Two of the groups were new and needed assistance in setting up their utilization control and review programs.

Early in 1985, Dr. Bergan primarily helped the nine IPAs set up their UR program and develop an HMO-wide peer review committee. This committee was made up of the presidents of the participating IPAs. In addition to performing peer review functions, this committee dealt with developing HMO utilization policies and implementing their IPA policies.

The Medicaid HMO Environment in Brown County

Public response to the HMO-AFDC program was mixed, as was reflected in a number of events occurring between mid-1985 and early 1986. First, in July 1985, a news article reported that five advocate groups felt the HMOs covering recipients of Aid to Families with Dependent Children/Medical Assistance should be required to be more thorough in their services. Then, in November 1985, a five-month-old girl died at home after allegedly being denied authorization to visit a hospital emergency room by an HMO pediatrician. The mother of the child filed an $8 million suit against the HMO, the hospital, and the pediatrician.

In January 1986, news media reported that the HMO-AFDC program was estimated to have saved the state $5.3 million in Medicaid costs in 1985, but many physicians felt that the result was a two-tiered medical system that denied the poor equal access to health care. In February 1986, an editorial appeared in the local paper challenging the state Medicaid director's statement that HMOs were "providing fine care to the poor." Later the same month another editorial stated the following:

> And it's also fair to wonder why certain contracts were renewed anyway when the state had evidence as early as late summer that they were not performing well. Sure, the new contracts specifically address quality-of-care issues, and at least some HMOs are on warning to shape up or suffer penalties, including possible loss of those contracts. Notice should have been served last fall, when the state could easily have demanded not just assurances but also hard evidence of correctives before any contracts were renewed. Because the state failed to use renewal as a club, it now has the heavy obligation to monitor the HMOs more closely than ever and be prepared to take its business elsewhere if commitments are not honored. "I intend to hold your feet to the fire," the state Medicaid director told HMO administrators. He had better bring out the matches.

The Independent Evaluation Agency Audit

In March 1985, an independent evaluator audited the internal QA programs of all HMOs participating in the initiative. The purpose was to verify the extent to which the internal QA programs of the individual HMOs were complete and functioning in ways consistent with the goal of ensuring adequate delivery of health care to enrollees.

The evaluators found that QA systems in most of the HMOs were not well developed. Many lacked basic structures and an organizational commitment to QA. Studies were often limited to physician services. Subcontracted care was not monitored. Complaint monitoring was often limited and not integrated into QA activities. Eight of the thirteen organizations had inadequate mechanisms for recording informal complaints. Serious efforts in disease prevention, health promotion, and health maintenance services were seen at only a few of the HMOs. Only three had written QA plans. Two had adequate-to-good QA studies underway. Increased staff commitment to QA has recommended for ten of the organizations. Time allotted to the medical director was insufficient to develop strong QA programs. In only three organizations was the evaluation staff able to identify a medical director actively involved in a QA program. Twelve had a UR program concentrating primarily on the financial implications of resource utilization.

In 1985, Dr. Bergan was primarily interested in bringing inpatient utilization under control and developing UR procedures in the IPAs. The peer review committee was meeting on a regular monthly basis with representation from all participating IPAs.

The Healthrite provider network was expanded further in 1986. The peer review committee began developing utilization controls for outpatient services and procedures and developed a system to monitor drug utilization. The HMO bought and implemented a new management information system that enabled the HMO to produce detailed reports of individual physician practice patterns.

Dr. Bergan began to hear complaints from the IPA administrative leaders and individual physicians late in the summer of 1986. Many physicians were frustrated by their lower incomes and the perceived invasion of their individual practices. To complicate matters, Healthrite HMO began to convert from nonprofit to for-profit status. This depleted reserves, tightened cash flow, and increased pressure on the IPAs to control costs. Table 18.2 shows the effect of the change in status on the HMO's revenues and expense.

During the fall of 1985 and throughout 1986, the HMOs began to feel pressure from the public media and advocate groups alleging that substandard care was being delivered to Medicaid recipients. Scrutiny of HMOs intensified after an infant allegedly died because Medqual (another Medicaid HMO) refused access to care in an emergency room. The legislative public hearing on MEI and continuing negative press reports forced Healthrite to examine its on-call system and memorandum of understanding with the ambulance companies and emergency room physicians. In addition, Dr. Bergan began a review of Healthrite's QA activities. To his dismay, he found that only four of the nine IPAs had conducted any QA studies.

The next week a ranking officer of one of their largest union clients scheduled a meeting to talk about the press reports regarding alleged substandard care delivered by HMOs. Many union members were upset that they had been forced into an HMO and wanted to reexamine this in the upcoming contract. Dr. Bergan resolved to improve the QA activities in Healthrite. He called a staff meeting to begin development of a

Table 18.2   Healthrite HMO, Revenue and Expense Summary

	1985 (Nonprofit)	1986 (For-profit)
Revenue		
Commercial premiums	$46,800,000	$61,272,000
Medicaid premiums	10,920,000	12,870,000
Other	532,000	601,000
Total revenue	58,252,000	74,743,000
Expenditures		
Medical and hospital	52,426,800	68,400,125
Administration	3,669,876	6,612,008
Total expenditures	56,096,676	75,012,133
Net income	2,155,324	(269,133)
Average number of commercial enrollees	60,000	72,000
Average number of Medicaid enrollees	14,000	16,500

plan for a comprehensive centralized QA program. The staff meeting produced a detailed list of needed resources and an outline of an implementation timetable. He put the items on the agenda for the upcoming peer review committee and sent a draft copies to the officers of all the IPA associations.

Dr. Bergan soon realized how difficult it would be to implement this plan. The first call he received was from one of the HMO physicians, Dr. Fesko, who complained, "Not only do we have to put up with all of your paperwork, but now you want to come into our offices, review our records, and tell us how to practice medicine! This is the last straw! If Healthrite doesn't get more physician-friendly, our IPA might take our enrollees to other HMOs."

That same day Dr. Bergan received three other calls during which he heard phrases like "big brotherism," "the straw that may break the camel's back," "approaching socialized medicine," "traitor" (this was from someone he had practiced with for ten years), and "corporate sellout."

Not all the calls were negative. Dr. Lindbloom, of St. Patrick's IPA, called to give support. St. Patrick's had a fairly well-developed QA program. Dr. Bergan told Dr. Lindbloom about the negative feedback. In response, Dr. Lindbloom said, "I think your problem is those fines you are handing out. I heard Dr. Spears got fined over $2,000 on one case for inappropriate length of stay. The MD names are on those individual physician practice profiles. There is a lot of negative peer pressure. The IPAs are distrustful of your QA program."

Many primary care physicians in Brown County belonged to HMOs. Some pediatricians and obstetricians belonged to as many as six competing HMOs. This meant that many physicians were dealing with different sets of HMO rules and regulations regarding practice patterns. Each HMO seemed to be waiting for the other to be the leader. He also feared that some IPAs would move into another HMO rather than be "harassed" by quality monitoring.

At the state HMO association meeting, Dr. Bergan had lunch with Dr. Phil Koch, the medical director at Medqual HMO. Dr. Bergan learned that Dr. Koch faced the same IPA and physician resistance to QA initiatives in his HMO. Dr. Bergan was surprised and laughingly said, "But *your* HMO is one of the HMOs that my IPAs say is more physician-friendly!"

Dr. Bergan felt the real issues were monetary issues and utilization control procedures. He saw the decentralized system as fragmented and inefficient. The proposed centralized QA program caught the wrath of the physicians because it was the last of a series of controls. The four IPA presidents who had contacted Dr. Bergan regarding this newest proposal stated that they were going to poll their membership to determine if they wanted to pursue contract renewal with Healthrite.

The Second Audit

In mid-1986, the evaluation agency forwarded the results of their second audit to Healthrite. The audit stated that Healthrite had not been in contract compliance on several issues. Healthrite did not have a functioning multidisciplinary broad-based committee. The model QA plan was still in draft form. It had not been approved by the IPAs or the Healthrite board of directors. Plans for hiring additional QA staff had not materialized. The QA program at Healthrite had a heavy utilization control and UR emphasis. QA studies and surveys conducted in 1985 and 1986 were minimal and lacking in both breadth and depth. The evaluation agency gave the Healthrite QA program the following overall assessment:

> Given the current organizational unrest, the reported resistance to the new QA program, the developmental stage of the QA program, and the past emphasis on utilization control and UR activities, it is recommended that the QA program of this HMO be closely monitored. This HMO

should be required to submit regular reports to the state Medicaid agency on the progress it is making in improving its QA program.

The report went on to recommend that the QA program be improved by using encounter data for problem identification, better integration of informal complaint reports and the QA program, monitoring of possible underservice, and development of formal tie-in to the QA programs of their major subcontractor hospitals. In addition, the HMO needed to improve the number of and methodology for QA studies, its feedback to subcontractors, and its monitoring of corrective action plans.

A few days after receiving the audit report, the executive director, Lars Hargrove, called Dr. Bergan and said, "You know, I've been looking at this audit report and the contract requirements, and I think we should call their bluff. This contract is ambiguous. We should challenge it and state that we are in contract compliance and that our UR program focuses primarily on quality issues and not on financial issues."

The HMO administration and board of directors were concerned about the report and looked to Dr. Bergan to take the necessary actions to correct the cited deficiencies. There were several options, but which would be best?

Boarder Babies

Beverly Hills and David A. Kindig, M.D.

Paula Valdez, M.D., arrived at her desk Tuesday morning following a 7:00 breakfast meeting with a gay rights committee protesting the city's lack of response to the AIDS crisis. At the top of her in-basket, she found a letter from the U.S. District Court informing her of a lawsuit filed against the city of Metropole, her office, and the Commissioner's office at the Department of Social Services. Dr. Valdez was the president of the Metropole Health and Hospitals Corporation (HHC). The HHC was incorporated by an act of the state legislature as a public benefit corporation with its own board of directors, and was charged with operating the city's municipal hospital system. The system included 16 hospitals, five neighborhood family care centers, and several other off-site programs.

The lawsuit had been filed by Maria Calvert on behalf of the Benefits to Children Organization, Baby Boy Norden, and Baby Girl Miller. Both children were "boarder babies" in one of Metropole's municipal hospitals. The suit charged that the city's failure to discharge hospitalized children and place them with families on a timely basis violated the children's constitutional rights, damaged their growth patterns, and injured their intellectual, social, and emotional development.

Dr. Valdez was aware that the census of these children had doubled over the past year. The boarder babies were defined as infants who were under the jurisdiction of Children's Services (CS) in the Metropole Department of Social Services (DSS), and had remained in the hospital ten or more days after being medically cleared for discharge. Children's Services was a division of the DSS, the city agency responsible for welfare services. It had the responsibility for investigating allegations of child abuse and neglect and overseeing placement of children in foster care. Fifty-five nonprofit city agencies worked with Children's Services. Sometimes Children's Services put a "hold" on these infants for various reasons. Some were waiting for decisions by the court as to appropriate disposition; others were determined to be appropriate for foster care placement and were waiting for hospital social workers and discharge planners to find appropriate placements. There was a critical shortage of foster care placements, especially for infants. It was the policy of HHC not to discharge any patient without an appropriate discharge plan.

The shortage of foster care options appeared to be due to a number of factors. More babies were being abandoned by their parents. There had been a 30 percent increase in one year in reported abuse and neglect cases due to recent changes in state law. More babies were being born with the AIDS virus, and many were born with complications resulting from their mothers' drug addiction. More women were seeking daytime jobs out of the home and were unavailable to be foster parents. The pool of foster parents was further limited by the fact that DSS social workers abided by an unwritten policy of placing babies with families of the same ethnic background in homes within the city. Therefore, many babies ended up staying in HHC and nonmunicipal hospitals for weeks and even months past the date of medical clearance for discharge.

The majority of the boarder babies did not receive parental visits. The fact that hospitals or institutions were not the optimal sites for infant stimulation and development was well documented. The detrimental effects on the intellectual and social development of children raised in institutions with ever-changing caregivers and limited social stimulation was found to cause problems such as abnormal social behaviors, impaired intellectual functioning, and retarded language capabilities.

Dr. Valdez asked her staff assistant to conduct an up-to-date census of boarder babies in each HHC hospital and to try to determine the reasons for their status. Dr. Valdez would use this data in a meeting with the DSS commissioner the following week. The statistics her assistant collected are shown in Table 19.1.

The following Wednesday morning, while Dr. Valdez was riding the bus to work, a headline in the City section of the daily newspaper popped out at her: "CITY HAS NO EXCUSE TO JAIL BABIES." The inflammatory article suggested that the city treated its animals more humanely than its babies. It cited the case of a zoo being closed so animals wouldn't be caged, and pointed out that the city was still caging

Table 19.1 Summary Statistics Survey of Children in HHC Hospitals at Least 10 Days Past Medical Clearance Awaiting SSC Placement (1/1/84–6/30/84 and 1/1/86–6/30/86)

Time Period	Age (years)	Number (%)	Average Length of Stay		
			Pre–Medical Clearance (days)	Post–Medical Clearance (days)	Total (days)
1/1/84–6/30/84	0–1	62 (52%)	20	24	44
	1–18	58 (48%)	31	63	94
		120			
1/1/86–6/30/86	0–1	209 (70%)	21	30	51
	1–18	91 (30%)	15	25	40
		300			

babies in hospitals. It criticized the city for making the foster care process a slow and burdensome one, with innocent babies being the losers.

Not one-half hour after she arrived at her office, she received a call from the Deputy Mayor, David Marshall. Marshall was the city's representative for issues affecting health and human services. He said, "The City is very upset about this boarder baby issue. You know this is an election year! This issue can have very serious political ramifications if we don't take immediate action!" Dr. Valdez explained the steps she was taking and her timetable. Marshall said she would have to work faster and that he would convene a meeting of the relevant agency heads that afternoon to give them their marching orders.

Dr. Valdez called her friend, Sam Epstein, M.D., the chief of pediatrics at one of the municipal hospitals mentioned in the news article. Dr. Epstein confirmed that there indeed was a baby born there who had just celebrated his first birthday. Since he had learned to walk, they had placed a metal net over his crib so he would not fall out onto the floor. His mother, a cocaine user, had abandoned him at birth. Placement had been very difficult, so he lived on the fourth floor of the hospital. The nurses tried their best to give the baby love and attention, but Dr. Epstein was very frank about the child's lack of toys and other stimulation, as well as the lack of attention he received from nurses who, because of the nursing shortage, needed to spend more time delivering basic nursing care to a large pediatric ward.

The next call was to Joe Piper, the DSS commissioner. When it

5-p0 nuxf -lrg-4u+df-s

came to the politics of the city's welfare programs, and Children's Services in particular, Joe Piper was described as a "fire fighter trying to put out a volcano." He had also received a call from the deputy mayor that morning. He indicated to Dr. Valdez that it took two to four months to do a thorough investigation of a foster care placement. "State regulations require that home studies be quite thorough," he said. "Sacrificing a thorough check is unconscionable." He said that the agency was willing to do whatever it could with its limited resources, people, and funds. Dr. Valdez explained her plan and suggested they meet as soon as the staff was able to get some information together.

On Thursday morning, the HHC board met at its regular time. Dr. Valdez presented the situation and told them of her response to the extensive publicity. She explained that the issue needed some immediate attention as well as short- and long-term strategies. The media was taking HHC to task for the crisis. The deputy mayor wanted a plan of action. Board member Fred Green, a community organizer and supporter of the challenger in the upcoming election, was outraged that there were allegations of over 100 babies boarding in hospitals at the present. "Mismanagement is what it is! The city had better come up with more money to hire more nurses to take care of these babies. The mayor is going to pay for this one!"

Dr. Betty Tregoning, the commissioner of the Department of Mental Health, spoke up next. "Look Fred, let's try to remove this issue from the political scene. We have an interagency problem here. On one hand, we have babies born with medical needs. But after those needs are stabilized, everyone agrees they should be moved out of the hospitals to foster care as soon as possible. What do you think about this, Joe?"

Joe Piper responded, "Clearly, this issue effects all our departments. Children's Services needs the time to examine the impact upon the family and the community. Where and how to place these babies is an issue for us if the mom is unable to care for the infant. We are extremely short on foster care placements. The agencies that make placements are "maxed out." Because of the press, we've had some phone calls from single working women who are willing to become foster mothers, and from people in neighboring cities. But they will all have to be processed, and some may not fall within our guidelines for foster parents."

"This is a Pandora's Box," said Dr. Anna Blake, a pediatrician and member of the board. "Ideally, we would like to find pregnant moms with drug problems in early pregnancy, so we could help them get treatment and focus on prevention issues. But when a mother comes into labor admitting to some drug use during pregnancy, staff automatically test the newborn's blood for drugs. If any show up, they are required to notify Children's Services, who will take custody of the baby. I know that the American Civil Liberties Union demands that a pregnant woman has civil rights and that what she does with her body while pregnant is her choice. But don't we have a responsibility to protect those babies? And what about the dollars the taxpayers are shelling out for neonatal intensive care costs?"

"These issues are extremely complicated," said Colleen O'Brien, a citizen member of the HHC board. "What about the financing for such a prevention program? Betty, is there any funding available in your agency? Drug abuse is a national problem. Surely the extra funding Congress is loosening up will be made available to deal with pregnant drug users. It seems to me that more social services dollars will also need to be tapped for foster care."

"I have heard talk about using volunteers to work with these babies," said Gretchen Maier, a board member with strong connections to the city unions. "I will strongly oppose any plan that takes jobs away from HHC or Children's Services workers!"

Deputy Mayor, David Marshall, who was also a member of the board, was a smooth and a competent political analyst. The city's financial position was especially tough this year due to a cap in tax revenue. The HHC's budget was nearly $2.3 billion, of which $500 million came from general tax levy support. Although the corporation's funding had not been cut by the same percentage as most other city agency budgets in the last budget round, the facilities were under pressure to maximize collection efforts and to stay within very tight budgets this year. The mayor was under intense political pressure to increase funding for police, education, and bridge replacement. The welfare roles had expanded and the DSS had already gotten some new dollars for foster care expansion, although apparently not enough. Maybe the DSS and HHC programs were flawed. Negotiations with city unions, including the hospital workers, were certain to require substantial increases.

Mr. Blomquist, the chair of the HHC board, spoke out. "You know, I am not pleased with HHC's fiscal relationship to Metropole. Hospital-generated revenues continue to be returned to city coffers. Because the hospital system collects much of what it spends, in contrast to most city agencies, it should be given greater fiscal autonomy and encouraged to develop a system that rewards good management. The increased patient census has generated new revenues for the city, and at the same time the amount of cash collected has risen steadily over the last few years. Ironically, few benefits have accrued to the hospitals from these increases. I don't think HHC should be asked to pay for solving a problem that, in my opinion, it didn't cause and can't solve alone."

"This all may be true, Mr. Blomquist," David Marshall said. "I can assure you that the city is willing to discuss all the available alternatives. I will be glad to take these issues back to the other city officials. Dr. Valdez, Dr. Tregoning, Mr. Piper, and I will be reviewing these issues later this week to generate a plan of options for review by the city administration."

Learning through the Case Method

Anthony R. Kovner

A challenge for many graduate programs in health services management is bridging the gap between theory and skills and their application to health services organizations. Part of the problem lies in the difficulty of attracting and retaining skilled teachers who can integrate perspectives and apply concepts across disciplines when responding to managerial problems and opportunities.

A second challenge is to prepare graduates to communicate effectively, in writing and orally, and to assist them in working effectively in groups. This includes helping students to assess the effects of their personalities or behavioral styles on others. Is the student perceived as abrasive, wishy-washy, manipulative? Are students aware of how others interpret not only their words but their tone and body language?

Students in graduate programs of health services management need to understand their own values and those of others who differ in educational background, political and religious orientation, clinical experience, or because of the careers and orientations of their parents and siblings.

A *case* is a description of a situation or problem actually faced by a manager and that requires analysis, decision, and planning of a course of action. A decision may be to delay a decision, and a planned course of action may be to take no action. A case takes place in time. A case

Reprinted from *Health Services Management: A Book of Cases*, 3d ed., edited by A. R. Kovner and D. Neuhauser (Ann Arbor, MI: Health Administration Press, 1989), with permission, Health Administration Press.

must have an issue. As McNair says, "There must be a question of what should somebody do, what should somebody have done, who is to blame for the situation, what is the best decision to be made under the circumstances."[1] A case represents selection from a situation; it represents selection by the casewriter.

The case method involves class discussion, guided by a teacher so that students can diagnose and define important problems in a situation, acquire competence in developing useful alternatives to respond to such problems, and improve judgment in selecting action alternatives. Students learn to diagnose constraints and opportunities faced by the manager and how to overcome constraints, given limited time and dollars.

Teachers can transmit great quantities of data to students more effectively and certainly more efficiently by lecture. Teachers are assumed to be correct in their presentation of facts, and students transcribe key points of the lectures and transmit them back to the teacher at examination time.

In a case course, the teacher's job is to engage the students in a management simulation so that they can think independently, communicate effectively, and defend their opinions logically with reference to underlying assumptions and values. Often there are no right answers to a case because, in dealing with issues, there are at least two sides to every question.

It is often difficult for students to adjust to a classroom in which there is no authority figure, no lecture from which to take notes, and a teacher who withholds information, at least until the class discussion has ended. Some students find it irritating to have to listen to their peers when they are paying to learn what the teacher has to say.

In a case course, students learn how to use information at the point of decision. Many students dislike "putting themselves on the line" when they are "only" students saying what they think. Although there are no "right" answers, students quickly learn in a case course that there are many "wrong" answers in terms of faulty logic or assumptions that are challenged or contradicted by their peers. Students fear looking foolish and being downgraded by the teacher. And they must pass the course.[2] Students should consider such exposure to be at low cost relative to the benefit they'll receive by being mature and skillful after graduation and in the professional environment. It is hoped that they will gain judgment and learn how to behave and communicate their opinions to others.

As Cantor says, "You don't learn from anybody else's experience or from your own experience unless you go through the experience to learn."[3] This is what the case method has to offer students—an experience in learning that involves testing their opinions and conclusions against the reality of the cases and the judgment of peers and teachers.

How do cases bridge the gap between theory and skills and their application by managers? Problems faced by health services managers do not come neatly packaged as separate questions of statistics, economics, organizational theory, or policy analysis. Rather, they are organizational, multidisciplinary problems, sometimes difficult to define as well as to resolve. Problems may include the negotiation of a new contract with the chief of radiology, appropriate response to patient complaints, or responsibility for quality assurance in relation to a surgeon's poor performance.

Student performance in a case course is typically assessed by their participation in class and their written analysis of case materials. Teachers sometimes cannot spend sufficient time on student evaluation, which may be partially corrected by allowing peer evaluation as well. Often teachers ask students to collaborate on complex cases or to evaluate each other's performance. Students should be told if their style or mannerisms interfere with their presentation or the way they are perceived by others.

In a case course, students are often asked to adopt the perspectives of certain characters in the case, to play certain roles. To deny someone something or to persuade them to do something requires an understanding of the person, their needs, and their perceptions of the decision maker. Role playing can promote a better understanding of viewpoints that may otherwise seem irrational, given a student's prior understanding of what should be done in a particular situation. Students can better understand their own values and underlying assumptions when their opinions are challenged by peers and teachers.

To conclude, it is important to understand what a case is not and what the case method cannot teach. Cases are not real life—they present only part of a situation. Writing or explaining a case may be as difficult or more difficult than evaluating someone else's written case. Like many consultants, students can never see what would have happened if the case participants had followed their advice.

There are some aspects of management that can only be learned by managing. How else can one know when someone says one thing but means another? How else can one judge when, if ever, to confront or oppose a member of the ruling coalition when that member's behavior appears to threaten the long-range interests of the organization? Students and managers have to form and adopt their own value systems and make their own decisions. A case course can give students a better understanding of the nature of the roles they will be playing as managers— an understanding that can help them to manage better and even to excel.

Notes

1. Andrew R. Towl, *To Study Administration by Cases* (Boston: Graduate School of Business Administration, Harvard University, 1969), 67.
2. Ibid., 68.
3. Ibid., 155.

A Short History of the Case Method of Teaching

Karen Schachter Weingrod and Duncan Neuhauser

No doubt Teaching by example is as old as the first parent and child. In medicine it surely started with a healer, the first apprentice, and a patient. The ancient Greeks codified medical principles, rules, and laws. University education in medicine started about 800 years ago, focused on abstract principles and scholastic reasoning, and was removed from practicality. By 1750 in England, the professions aspired to gentleman status.[1] The goldheaded cane of the English physician was the clear symbol that his hands were not expected to touch patients, unlike apothecaries and barber surgeons. Later, the American sociologist Thorstein Veblen, in *The Theory of the Leisure Class*, used the example of the cane as a symbol that a gentleman need not work with his hands.[2] In the late 1700s in France, medical education moved into hospitals, or "the clinic," where patients in large numbers could be observed, autopsies performed, and the physiological state linked back to the patients' signs and symptoms.[3] This was one step in the departure from abstract medical theorizing in universities (often about the four humors), which had no proven bearing on actual disease processes.

Education in law also became increasingly abstract, conveyed through erudite lectures that were built upon theoretical constructs and logically well reasoned. The professor spoke and the student memo-

---

Reprinted from *Health Services Management: A Book of Cases*, 3d ed., edited by A. R. Kovner and D. Neuhauser (Ann Arbor, MI: Health Administration Press, 1989), with permission, Health Administration Press.

rized and recited, without much opportunity for practical experience or discussion. This had become the standard by the late 1850s. Thus, it is only by comparison with what went before it in universities that the case method of teaching is so unusual.

The historical development of the case method can be traced to Harvard University. Perhaps it is not surprising that this occurred in the United States rather than in Europe, with the American inclinations toward democratic equality, practicality, and positivism, and the lack of interest in abstract scholastic theorizing. The change started in 1870, when the president of Harvard University, Charles William Eliot, appointed the obscure lawyer Christopher Columbus Langdell to be the dean of Harvard Law School. Langdell believed law to be a science. In his own words, "Law considered as a science, consists of certain principles or doctrines. To have such a mastery of these as to be able to apply them with constant faculty and certainty to the ever-tangled skein of human affairs, is what constitutes a good lawyer; and hence to acquire that mastery should be the business of every earnest student of the law."[4]

The specimens needed for the study of Langdell's science of law were judicial opinions as recorded in books and stored in libraries. He accepted the science of law, but he turned the learning process back to front. Instead of giving a lecture that would define a principle of law and give supporting examples of judicial opinions, he gave the students the judicial opinions without the principle and, by use of a Socratic dialogue, extracted from the students in the classroom the principles that would make sense out of the cases. The student role was now active rather than passive. Students were subjected to rigorous questioning of the case material. They were asked to defend their judgments and to confess to error when their judgments were illogical. Although this dialectic was carried on by the professor and one or two students at a time, all the students learned and were on the edge of their seats, fearing or hoping to be called on next. The law school style that evolved puts the student under public pressure to reason quickly, clearly, and coherently in a way that is valuable in the courtroom or during negotiation. After a discouraging start, Langdell attracted such able instructors as Oliver Wendell Holmes, Jr. They carried the day, and now the case method of teaching is nearly universal in U.S. law schools.

The introduction of the case method of teaching to medicine is also known. A Harvard medical student of the class of 1901, Walter B. Cannon shared a room with Harry Bigelow, a third-year law student. The excitement with which Bigelow and his classmates debated the issues within the cases they were reading for class contrasted sharply with the passivity of medical school lectures. In 1900, discussing the value of the case method in medicine, Harvard President Charles Eliot described the earlier medical education as follows:

> I think it was thirty-five years ago that I was a lecturer at the Harvard Medical School for one winter; at that time lectures began in the school at eight o'clock in the morning and went on steadily till two o'clock—six mortal hours, one after the other of lectures, without a question from the professor, without the possibility of an observation by the student, none whatever, just the lecture to be listened to, and possibly taken notes of. Some of the students could hardly write.[5]

In December 1899, Cannon persuaded one of his istructors, G. L. Walton, to present one of the written cases from his private practice as an experiment. Walton printed a sheet with the patient's history and allowed the students a week to study it. The lively discussion that ensued in class made Walton an immediate convert.[6] Other faculty soon followed, including Richard C. Cabot.

Through the case method, medical students would learn to judge and interpret clinical data, to estimate the value of evidence, and to recognize the gaps in their knowledge—something that straight lecturing could never reveal. The case method of teaching allowed students to throw off passivity in the lecture hall and integrate their knowledge of anatomy, physiology, pathology, and therapeutics into a unified mode of thought.

As a student, Cannon wrote two articles about the case method in 1900 for the *Boston Medical and Surgical Journal* (later to become *The New England Journal of Medicine*).[7] He sent a copy of one of these papers to a famous clinician professor, Dr. William Osler of Johns Hopkins. Osler replied, "I have long held that the only possible way of teaching students the subject of medicine is by personal daily contact with cases, which they study not only once or twice, but follow systematically."[8] If a written medical case was interesting, a real live patient in the classroom could be memorable. Osler regularly introduced patients to his class and asked students to interview and examine the patient and discuss the medical problems involved. He would also send students to the library and laboratory to seek answers and report back to the rest of the class.[9] This was ideal teaching and Osler's students worshiped him, but with today's division of labor in medicine between basic science and clinical medicine, such a synthesis is close to impossible.

The 24 May 1900 issue of the *Boston Medical and Surgical Journal* was devoted to articles and comments about the case method of teaching written by Eliot, Cannon, Cabot, and others. In some ways it remains the best general discussion of the case method. This approach was adopted rapidly at other medical schools, and books of written cases quickly followed in neurology (1902), surgery (1904), and orthopedic surgery (1905).[10]

Walter Cannon went on to a distinguished career in medical research. Richard C. Cabot joined the medical staff of the Massachusetts General Hospital and published his first book of cases in 1906. (He also introduced the first social worker into a hospital.[11]) He was concerned with the undesirable separation of clinical physicians and pathologists. Too many diagnoses were turning out to be false at autopsy. To remedy this, Cabot began to hold his case exercises with students, house officers, and visitors.

Cabot's clinical/pathological conferences took on a stereotyped style that was eventually adopted in teaching hospitals throughout the world. First, the patient's history, symptoms, and test results were described. Then, an invited specialist would discuss the case, suggest an explanation, and give a diagnosis. Finally, the pathologist would present the autopsy or pathological diagnosis and questions would follow to elaborate points.

In 1915 Cabot sent written copies of his cases to interested physicians as "at home case method exercises." These became so popular that in 1923 the *Boston Medical and Surgical Journal* began to publish one per issue.[12] This journal has since changed its name to *The New England Journal of Medicine*, but the "Cabot Case Records" still appear with each issue.

A look at a current case in *The New England Journal of Medicine* will show how much the case method has changed since Christopher Columbus Langdell's original concept. The student or house officer is no longer asked to discuss the case; rather, it is experts who put their reputation on the line. They have the opportunity to demonstrate wisdom, but they can also be refuted in front of a large audience. Every physician in the audience probably makes mental diagnoses, but in general case presentations have become a more passive affair, more like traditional lectures.

Richard Cabot left the Massachusetts General Hospital to head the social relations (sociology, psychology, cultural anthropology) department at Harvard. He brought the case method with him, but it disappeared from use there by the time of his death in 1939.[13] The social science disciplines were concerned with theory building, hypothesis testing, and research methodology, and perhaps the case method was considered primitive to such unapplied pure scientists. The use of case method in the first two preclinical years of medical school also diminished, as clinical scientists came more and more to the fore with their laboratory work and research on physiology, pharmacology, biochemistry, and molecular biology. A return to a problem-solving focus in medical school is now being advocated by a task force of the American Association of Medical Colleges.

In 1908 the Harvard Business School was created as a department of Harvard's Graduate School of Arts and Sciences. It was initially criticized as merely a school for successful money making. There was an effort early on to teach through the use of written problems involving situations faced by actual business executives, presented in sufficient factual detail to enable students to develop their own decisions. The school's first book of cases, on marketing, was published in 1922 by Melvin T. Copeland.[14]

Today, nearly every class in the Harvard Business School is taught by the case method. In 1957 the Intercollegiate Case Clearing House was founded. Located on campus, it housed approximately 40,000 cases and added 1,000 to 1,200 new cases each year. Cases were also made available to other universities. The clearing house has since been renamed HBS Case Services and now limits itself to cases produced at the Harvard Business School.

Unlike the law school, where cases come directly from judicial decisions and are sometimes abbreviated by the instructor, and unlike the medical school, where the patient is the basis for the case, the business faculty and their aides must enter organizations to collect and compile their material. In doing so there is substantial editorial latitude. Here more than elsewhere the case writer's vision, or lack of it, defines the content of the case.

Unlike a pathologist's autopsy diagnosis, a business case is not designed to have a right answer. In fact, one never knows whether the business in question lives or dies. Rather, the cases are written in such a way as to split a large class (up to 80 students) into factions. The best cases are those that create divergent opinions. The professor becomes more of an orchestra leader than a source of truth. The professor's opinion or answer may never be made explicit. Following a discussion, a student's question as to what really happened or what should have been done may be answered with "I don't know," or "I think the key issues were picked up in the case discussion." Such hesitancy on the part of the instructor is often desirable. To praise or condemn a particular faction in the classroom can discourage future discussions.

The class atmosphere in a business school is likely to be less pressured than in a law school. Like a good surgeon, a good lawyer must often think very quickly, but unlike the surgeon the lawyer's thinking is demonstrated verbally and publicly. Lawyers must persuade by the power of logic rather than by force of authority. Business and management are different. Key managerial questions—What business are we in? or Who are our customers? or Where should we be ten years from now?—may take months or even years to answer.

The fact that the business manager's time frame reduces the pressure for immediate answers makes management education different from physician education in other ways. Physicians are required to absorb countless facts on anatomy, disease symptoms, and drug side effects. Confronted with 20 patients a day, the physician has no time to consult references and so must rely on memory instead. Managers can look up information because they have more time for decision making. Therefore, managerial education focuses more on problem-solving techniques than on memorization of data.

Not all business schools have endorsed the case method of teaching. The University of Chicago Business School, for example, rarely uses cases and instead focuses on teaching the science of economics, human behavior, and operations research. The faculty are concerned with theory building, hypothesis testing, statistical methodology, and the social sciences. Stanford Business School uses about half social sciences and half case method. Each school is convinced that its teaching philosophy is best and believes others to be misguided. Conceptually, the debate can be broken into two aspects: science versus professionalism, and active versus passive learning.

There is little doubt that active student involvement in learning is better than passively listening to lectures. The case method is one of many approaches to increasing student participation. However, only a skilled instructor can stimulate a lively discussion—for example, by social sciences students on the theoretical assumptions, methodological problems, and use or abuse of statistical analysis in an *American Journal of Sociology* assignment.

Academic science is not overly concerned with the practical problems of the world, but professionals are and professional education should be. The lawyer, physician, and manager cannot wait for perfect knowledge. They have to make decisions in the face of uncertainty. Science can help with these decisions to varying degrees. To the extent that scientific theories have the power to predict and explain, they can be used by professionals. In the jargon of statistics: the higher that percentage of variance explained, the more useful the scientific theory, the smaller the role for clinical or professional judgment, and the greater the role for case method teaching as opposed to, for example, mathematical problem solving.

It can be argued that the professional will always be working at the frontier of the limits of scientific prediction. When science is the perfect predictor, then often the problem is solved, or the application is delegated to computers or technicians, or, as in some branches of engineering, professional skills focus on the manipulation of accurate but complex mathematical equations.

Scientific medicine now understands smallpox so well that it no longer exists. Physicians spend most of their time on problems that are not solved: cancer, heart disease, or the common complaints of living that bring most people to doctors. In management, the budget cycle, personnel position control, sterile operating room environment, and maintenance of the business office ledgers are handled routinely by organizational members and usually do not consume the attention of the chief executive officer. In law, the known formulations become the "boiler plate" of contracts.

The debate among business schools over the use of cases illustrates the difference in beliefs about the power of the social sciences in the business environment. Teaching modes related to science and judgment will always be in uneasy balance with each other, shifting with time and place. A few innovative medical schools have moved away from the scientific lectures in the preclinical years and toward a case problem-solving mode (e.g., the University of Limburg in Maastricht, Holland). On the other side of the coin, a quiet revolution is being waged in clinical reasoning. The principles of statistics, epidemiology, and economics, filtered through the techniques of decision analysis, cost-effectiveness analysis, computer modeling, and artificial intelligence, are making the Cabot Case Record approach obsolete for clinical reasoning. Scientific methods of clinical reasoning are beginning to replace aspects of professional or clinical judgment in medicine.[15]

This does not mean that the professional aspect of medicine will be eliminated by computer-based science. Rather, the frontiers, the unknown areas calling for professional judgment, will shift to new areas such as the development of socioemotional rapport with patients—what used to be called "the bedside manner."

The cases in this book are derived from the business school style of case teaching. As such, they do not give answers. The cases can be used to apply concepts such as matrix organization or cost control analysis to practical problems. However, although the concepts (scientific theory seems too strong a term to apply to them) may help solve these case problems, they will not yield one right answer. They all leave much room for debate.

Notes

1. H. J. Cook, *The Decline of the Old Medical Regime in Stuart London* (Ithaca: Cornell University Press, 1986).

2. T. Veblen, *The Theory of the Leisure Class* (1899; reprinted New York; Mentor, 1953).

3. M. Foucault, *The Birth of the Clinic* (New York: Vintage, 1973).

4. C. C. Langdell, *Cases and Contracts (1871), cited in The Law at Harvard*, by A. E. Sutherland (Cambridge, MA: Harvard University Press, 1967), 174.

5. C. Eliot, "The Inductive Method Applied to Medicine," *Boston Medical and Surgical Journal* 142, no. 22 (May 24, 1900): 557.

6. S. Benison, A. Clifford Barger, and E. L. Wolfe, *Walter B. Cannon, The Life and Times of a Young Scientist* (Cambridge, MA: Harvard University Press, 1987), 65–75, 417–18.

7. W. B. Cannon, "The Case Method of Teaching Systematic Medicare," *The Boston Medical and Surgical Journal* 142, no. 2 (January 11, 1900): 31–36; and "The Case System in Medicine," 142, no. 22 (May 24, 1900): 563–64.

8. Benison, Barger, and Wolfe, *Walter B. Cannon*, 66.

9. A. M. Chesney, *The Johns Hopkins Hospital and the Johns Hopkins University School of Medicine*, Vol. II 1893–1905 (Baltimore: The Johns Hopkins Press, 1958), 125–28.

10. Benison, Barger, and Wolfe, *Walter B. Cannon*, 418.

11. Although not the first hospital-based social worker to work with Cabot, his best known social worker colleague was Walter Cannon's sister, Ida Cannon. See Benison, Barger, and Wolfe, *Walter B. Cannon*, 145.

12. These cases start October 25, 1923.

13. P. Buck, ed. *The Social Sciences at Harvard* (Boston, MA: Harvard University Press, 1965).

14. For more on the history of the case method of teaching managers, see R. Penchansky, *Health Services Administration: Policy Cases and the Case Method* (Boston, MA: Harvard University Press, 1968), 395–453.

15. The proposal to increase the problem-solving content of medical education is found in Association of American Medical Colleges, *Graduate Medical Education: Proposals for the Eighties* (Washington, DC: AAMC, 1980); also reprinted as a supplement in *Journal of Medical Education* 56, no. 9 (September 1981, part 2).

List of Contributors

Alan R. Altman, M.D., M.S., FACP, is in the private practice of gastroenterology in Palm Springs, California. He was Chairman of the Department of Medicine at Desert Hospital from 1982 until 1987 and served in the U.S. Army from 1974 until 1976. He received his medical degree from New York Medical College in 1971, and did an internship, residency, and gastroenterology fellowship at Mount Sinai Hospital in New York City between 1971 and 1974, and between 1976 and 1978. He received his master's degree in administrative medicine from the University of Wisconsin–Madison in 1992.

Fred J. Barten, M.H.A., is Executive Vice President and Chief Operating Officer of Oakwood Health Services Corporation in Dearborn, Michigan. He earned his graduate degree at the University of Michigan. He has worked in hospital administration since 1968.

E. A. Bonfils-Roberts, M.D., is Chief of Chest Surgery at St. Vincent's Hospital and Medical Center, New York City. He received his medical degree from the University of Buenos Aires in 1962 and his training at Duke University, George Washington University, St. Vincent's Hospital and Medical Center, and the Mayo Graduate School of Medicine in Rochester, Minnesota. He is board certified in thoracic and cardiac surgery and holds a certificate of special qualifications in vascular surgery. In 1990 he received a Master of Science degree in health management from New York University. He has been affiliated with St. Vincent's Hospital and Medical Center since 1971 and is Assistant Clinical Professor of Surgery at New York University School of Medicine.

Scott A. Braucht, M.B.A., is a management consultant and principal at Smith & Gesteland, CPAs/Business Consultants, in Madison, Wisconsin.

He earned his M.B.A. in management and marketing at the University of Wisconsin–Madison. Previously, he worked as Manager of Operations and as Director of Provider Relations and Member Services for one of Wisconsin's largest health maintenance organizations. He is also a lecturer in the University of Wisconsin–Madison Administrative Medicine Program and serves on the school board in Verona, Wisconsin.

Richard M. Carr, M.D., M.S., practices clinical oncology/hematology at Quisling Clinic in Madison, Wisconsin. Since 1984 he has had a number of managerial responsibilities in the clinic and hospital. He received his medical degree at Stanford University School of Medicine in 1965. Dr. Carr did an internship at Montefiore Hospital in New York, a residency in internal medicine at the University of Michigan Hospital in Ann Arbor, Michigan, a fellowship in hematology at Simpson Memorial Institute at the University of Michigan (1968–1970), and a fellowship in clinical oncology at the University of Michigan Hospital (1970). He earned a Master of Science degree in administrative medicine at the University of Wisconsin–Madison in 1983.

Martin Cherkasky, M.D., is a co-chairman of the New York State Advisory Committee on Physician Recredentialing and the chairman of the Advisory Board to the Office of Chief Medical Examiner of New York City. He is also a consultant to Montefiore Medical Center and to the board of trustees of Montefiore Medical Center in The Bronx, New York. He served as the chief executive officer at Montefiore Medical Center for 30 years. He received his medical degree in 1936 from Temple University Medical School in Philadelphia. Dr. Cherkasky began his affiliation with Montefiore Hospital in 1937 as an assistant resident. He served in the Medical Corps of the armed forces from 1940 until 1946 and returned to Montefiore Hospital in 1945 as a Fellow in Medicine. He occupied various positions at the hospital until assuming the role of chief executive officer in 1951. He was elected to the Institute of Medicine in 1977.

Kenneth C. Cummings, M.D., FACPE, is Vice President for Medical Affairs at Saint Joseph Health Center in Kansas City, Missouri. He is board certified in pathology and medical management and has practiced medicine for 22 years in military, private practice, academic, and community settings. Beyond practicing pathology, he has been an academic department chairman, hospital medical director, and associate dean for clinical affairs. Currently, he is chairman of the editorial review board for *Physician Executive* and a director of the American Board of Medical Management. He received his medical degree from George Washington University in 1969.

Don E. Detmer, M.D., is Professor of Surgery, Professor of Business Administration, and Vice President for Health Sciences at the University of Virginia in Charlottesville, Virginia. A native of Kansas, he received his medical degree from the University of Kansas and took his surgical training at Duke University, Johns Hopkins University, and the National Institutes of Health. He studied health policy at the Institute of Medicine, National Academy of Sciences, and at the Harvard Business School. He then joined the faculty of the University of Wisconsin–Madison, where he created and directed programs in administrative medicine and peripheral vascular surgery and received a Chancellor's Distinguished Teaching Award in 1979. He served as Vice President of Health Sciences at the University of Utah before going to the University of Virginia. He is a member of the Institute of Medicine and the board of directors of the Association for Health Services Research.

James S. Emrich, M.P.H., is an independent management consultant focusing on the management and governance of not-for-profit organizations. He previously served as the executive vice president and chief operating officer of a behavioral science technology firm. He has also served as a chief financial officer and in senior management in a variety of health care settings, including ten years at the University of Pennsylvania Medical Center.

J. Richard Gaintner, M.D., is the president and chief executive officer of the New England Deaconess Hospital and its parent company, NEDH Corporation, in Boston, Massachusetts. He received his medical degree in 1962 from Johns Hopkins University School of Medicine and his undergraduate degree from Lehigh University in Pennsylvania. Prior to joining Deaconess in August 1989, he was the president and chief executive officer at Albany Medical Center in New York. From 1981 until 1983, he served as vice president and deputy director of Johns Hopkins Hospital in Baltimore. At Johns Hopkins, he also was the associate dean for administration in the school of medicine from 1977 until 1980. Prior to his tenure at Johns Hopkins, he was vice president for medical affairs at New Britain General Hospital in Connecticut and held a number of positions with the University of Connecticut School of Medicine from 1967 until 1975.

Carl J. Getto, M.D., is Vice Dean, Associate Dean for Clinical Affairs, and Associate Professor (CHS) in the Department of Psychiatry at the University of Wisconsin Medical School in Madison, Wisconsin. He received his medical degree from Loyola University Stritch School of Medicine in Chicago in 1972 and did a residency in psychiatry (1972–75) at the University of Colorado Medical Center, where he was a chief resident and teaching fellow in the Psychiatric Liaison Division (1974–75). He received a master's degree in management in 1991 from the Kellogg School of Business at Northwestern University in Evanston, Illinois. He was Director of the University of Wisconsin Pain Treatment Program from 1982 until 1987 and Director of Psychiatric Consultation Service at the University of Wisconsin Hospital and Middleton VA Hospital from 1979 until 1983. Prior to his affiliation with the department of psychiatry at the University of Wisconsin, which began in 1979, he was an assistant professor at the University of Colorado Medical Center in Denver, Colorado.

Beverly Hills, M.A., is a registered nurse at the University of Wisconsin Hospital and Clinics, Department of Psychiatry. She received her master's degree in public policy and administration, specializing in health services, from the University of Wisconsin–Madison in 1987. She has worked as a nurse in private and public settings, and has been active in political activities in South Dakota and Wisconsin. She has served as an elected Dane County Board Supervisor since 1986.

Robert B. Klint, M.D., M.H.A., FACPE, is President and Chief Executive Officer of SwedishAmerican Hospital and Corporation in Rockford, Illinois. SwedishAmerican is a midwestern health services network that operates two hospitals, physician group practices, a managed care organization, and a regional provider services network. Dr. Klint served as President of the American College of Physician Executives in 1987–1988. He earned degrees in economics from Brown University, in medicine from Northwestern University, and in hospital administration from the University of Minnesota. He is board certified in pediatrics and pediatric cardiology, which he practiced for eight years before entering medical management.

Jeffrey Kunz, M.D., M.A., is Chief Executive Officer of the Monona Grove Clinic and Clinical Associate Professor of Preventive Medicine and Rehabilitation Medicine at the University of Wisconsin Medical School in Madison, Wisconsin. He received his medical degree and a master's degree in health policy and administration in 1977 from the University of Wisconsin–Madison, and was a Scholl Fellow in Rehabilitation Medicine at Northwestern University Medical School in Chicago, Illinois. He has served in senior management positions with the American Medical Association, McGaw Medical Center of Northwestern University, the University of Wisconsin Medical School, and the State of Wisconsin Health Office.

Michael E. Kurtz, M.S., is a member of the core faculty of the American College of Physician Executives and was awarded honorary membership in the organization in 1985. He is a principal consultant to the National Institutes of Health and a faculty consultant for the American Group Practice Association, the Medical Group Management Association, the Group Health Association of America, and Healthcare Forum. He is President of the Training, Education, and Consultation Services Division of MD Resources, Inc., a physician recruitment and health care consulting firm in Miami, Florida. Mr. Kurtz completed his graduate work at the University of California at Berkeley and at the University of Southern California.

Abraham M. Lenobel, M.D., M.S., received his medical degree in 1956 from SUNY Medical School in Brooklyn and his master's degree in 1986 from New York University's Wagner School. He was a member of a medical board for 15 years and a hospital trustee for more than 7 years. He also served as a consultant to the New York State Department of Health on the last revision of the state hospital code, specifically, on the section on maternal and child care. He was in the private practice of obstetrics and gynecology for 22 years. For 14 years he occupied the Chair of a department similar to the one described in Case 1.

Karl Merkle, M.D., earned his medical degree at Heidelberg University in 1948, graduating magna cum laude. He emigrated to the United States in 1949, completed a three-year residency at Oakwood Hospital in Dearborn, Michigan, and has been in private practice since that time. He has been active at Oakwood Hospital as Chairman of the Department of Family Practice, and as Chief-Elect and Chief of Staff, for three years each. He was one of the founding directors of SelectCare. He is now Medical Affairs Consultant to Oakwood United Hospitals in Dearborn, Michigan.

Jerry Rose, M.B.A., is Corporate Vice President of Planning and Business Development for Oakwood Health Services Corporation in Dearborn, Michigan. Previously, he was Associate Director and Senior Lecturer in the Programs in Health Management, Department of Preventive Medicine, at the University of Wisconsin Medical School. During his 20-year affiliation with the University of Wisconsin, Mr. Rose taught courses in information systems, strategic planning, strategic management, statistics, quality of care, and consulting. He has also done consulting in the areas of medical management and information systems, and has been a coordinator of a joint venture between the University of Wisconsin–Madison and General Electric Medical Systems for seminars on technology management. Mr. Rose earned an M.B.A. in hospital administration from the University of Chicago and an M.B.A. in finance from Northwestern University.

Howard E. Rotner, M.D., FACPE, is Senior Vice President for Medical Affairs at AtlantiCare Medical Center in Lynn, Massachusetts. A graduate of Harvard Medical School, he is board certified in internal medicine and endocrinology. Prior to becoming the medical director at AtlantiCare in 1985, he was in private practice for 17 years, contributing significantly to the growth and success of his internal medicine group.

Carol Winkler Schramm, B.S., earned a Bachelor of Science degree in Business Administration/Marketing from Bradley University in Peoria, Illinois, in 1967. She has held a number of health care planning and management positions, and since 1985 she has been a researcher and project director for the Center for Health Policy and Program Evaluation at the University of Wisconsin–Madison. In this position, she was the project director for the Wisconsin HMO Medicaid Evaluation Project.

Barry M. Schultz, M.D., M.S., FACP, is a board-certified internist and formally trained geriatrician and is a Fellow of the American College of Physicians. He is Assistant Professor of Medicine and Gerontology and Director of the Program in Health Policy in the Center for Aging and Adult Development at the New York Medical College in Valhalla, New York. He is also Medical Director for Clinical and Administrative Affairs at the Ruth Taylor Geriatric and Rehabilitation Institute, a 400-bed long-term care facility that is the teaching nursing home for New York Medical College. He received his medical degree from Hahnemann University School of Medicine in Philadelphia in 1982. He received a Master of Science degree in health policy and management from the Wagner School of Public Policy's Advanced Management Program for Clinicians at New York University.

Richard L. Siegel, M.D., M.S., is board certified in both internal medicine and emergency medicine. For the past nine years, he has been Medical Director of the emergency department of a large teaching hospital in New Jersey. He received his medical degree in 1974 from Tufts University School of Medicine in Boston, Massachusetts, and did residencies in internal medicine at Framingham Union Hospital in Massachusetts and in emergency medicine at the Albert Einstein College of Medicine/Bronx Municipal Hospital in New York. He is a 1992 graduate of the Advanced Management Program for Clinicians (AMPC) at the Wagner School for Public Service of New York University, for which he earned a Master of Science degree in health care management.

Paul O. Simenstad, M.D., has been Medical Director of DeanCare HMO in Madison, Wisconsin, since 1983 and was an administrator with Dean Clinic prior to that time. He is also a clinical professor in the Department of Preventive Medicine at the University of Wisconsin–

Madison, where he has had a teaching appointment since 1965. He retired from private practice in general and internal medicine in July 1990 after more than 30 years in practice. He received his medical degree from the University of Rochester School of Medicine in 1954.

Timothy H. Sio, M.A., is Vice President of Professional Services for Meriter Hospital, Inc., a 517-bed acute care hospital in Madison, Wisconsin. He earned a Master of Arts degree in Business–Health Service Administration from the University of Wisconsin–Madison in 1988.

Paul M. Spilseth, M.D., M.S., is a family physician at St. Croix Valley Clinic in Stillwater, Minnesota. The clinic is a primary care, multispecialty group practice of 20 physicians. He is also Medical Director of Lakeview Hospital in Stillwater. He received his medical degree from the University of Minnesota in 1969. He completed an internship at St. Mary's Hospital in Duluth, Minnesota, a residency in family practice at the University of Oklahoma, and his Master of Science degree in administrative medicine from the University of Wisconsin–Madison in 1988.

Earl R. Thayer, B.A., earned a Bachelor of Arts in Journalism at the University of Wisconsin in 1947. He was employed by the State Medical Society of Wisconsin from 1947 until 1987, serving the last 15 years as Secretary–General Manager. He is a member of the board of directors of Blue Cross Blue Shield United of Wisconsin, United Wisconsin Services, Inc., and the Charitable Foundation of the State Medical Society.

Blake E. Waterhouse, M.D., M.B.A., has been President and CEO of Straub Clinic and Hospital in Honolulu, Hawaii, since 1990. Previously he was President and CEO of Physicians Plus Medical Group in Madison, Wisconsin (1987–1990). From 1965 until 1987 he was the first medical director of Jackson Clinic in Madison, Wisconsin. He received his medical degree from Indiana University School of Medicine in 1961 and completed a residency at Mayo Clinic and an internship at Iowa Methodist Hospital in Des Moines, Iowa. In 1988 he received an M.B.A. degree from the University of Wisconsin–Madison. He was a member of the Department of Internal Medicine at the University of Wisconsin School of Medicine from 1965 until 1990.

About the Editors

David A. Kindig, M.D., Ph.D., is Professor of Preventive Medicine and Director, Programs in Health Management, University of Wisconsin School of Medicine, Madison, Wisconsin. His graduate degrees are from the University of Chicago in 1968, and he served a residency in pediatrics and social medicine at Montefiore Hospital in the Bronx. As a medical student he was National President of the Student American Medical Association. His management positions include being the first Medical Director of the National Health Service Corps; Deputy Director, Bureau of Health Manpower, Department of Health, Education and Welfare; Executive Director, Montefiore Hospital and Medical Center; and Vice Chancellor for Health Sciences, University of Wisconsin–Madison. His research interests are in urban and rural health, primary care, administrative medicine, equity in health care, and international health. He currently serves as a commissioner of the Prospective Payment Assessment Commission, on the Agency for Health Care Policy and Research (AHCPR) Study Section for Research Dissemination, on the board of the Association of University Programs in Health Administration, on advisory boards of several rural research centers, and as Chair of the Wisconsin Area Health Education Center (AHEC) Advisory Committee.

Anthony R. Kovner, M.P.A., Ph.D., is Professor of Health Policy and Management at the Robert F. Wagner Graduate School of Public Service at New York University. He has served as Director of the Hospital Community Benefit Standards Program (HCBSP), a W. K. Kellogg Program to encourage implementation of systematic community benefit services programs for hospitals. He is a member of the board of trustees of Lutheran Medical Center. Before joining New York University, Dr. Kovner was Chief Executive Officer of the Newcomb Hospital of Vineland, New Jersey, and Senior Health Consultant to the United Auto Workers Union in Detroit, Michigan. Dr. Kovner is the author of *Really Managing: The Work of Effective CEOS in Large Health Organizations* as well as numerous books and articles about health services management. He received the 1991 Dean Conley Award from the American College of Healthcare Executives for his article "Improving Hospital Board Effectiveness: An Update," which was published in *Frontiers of Health Services Management* in Spring 1990. He is married with two children and lives in New York City.